SIBLING CAREGIVERS

How to Have a Life, Be Encouraged and Live Stress Free

OB NWAOGBE

OB NWAOGBE
TABLE OF CONTENTS

ACKNOWLEDGEMENTS iii
CHAPTER 1: OUR JOURNEY 1
CHAPTER 2: ENCOURAGEMENT 4
CHAPTER 3: WHO IS A SIBLING CAREGIVER? 10
CHAPTER 4: ACCEPTANCE 30
CHAPTER 5: THE CAREGIVERS' INCREDIBLE GIFTS, AND THE PEOPLE WHO DON'T APPRECIATE THEM 47
CHAPTER 6: RESOURCES 58
CHAPTER 7: ADVICE TO PARENTS 87
CHAPTER 8: DEALING WITH DISABILITIES IN AFRICAN COUNTRIES AND COMMUNITIES IN THE DIASPORA 115
CHAPTER 9: WHERE DO WE GO FROM HERE? 128
ABOUT THE AUTHOR 133
REFRENCES 134
INDEX 136

Sibling Caregiver
ACKNOWLEDGEMENTS

This book was inspired by my brother Anuforole O.Nwaogbe, fondly known to all as Rolly. Born with a developmental disability, being non-verbal and later on developing scoliosis is quite a bit for one person to handle. Despite it all, Rolly is always full of life and brings joy to everyone around him. Growing up with him taught me how to show compassion to people with disabilities, while empowering them to be independent individuals. But most importantly, it showed me patience and courage in the face of adversity.

Special thanks to my parents for bringing us into this world. To my mother who has been instrumental in shaping the way my life and that of Rolly's turned around for the better. To my dad who passed on on October 8, 2011; your tough love, resiliance and always being my biggest cheerleader has molded me into the woman I am today. To my family in Nigeria, as cliché as it might seem, you all gave a brand new meaning to "it takes a village."

Thank you to SEEC and Q-Care, the two caregiver organizations in the Washington D.C, area for taking on my brother as one of one of their own. I could not have made it through all these years as a caregiver without your help and support.

And finally to my family and friends, thank you for listening to me vent, cry, and accomodating my occasional hermit mode. Your love and understand has been getting Rolly and I through this journey!

CHAPTER 1: OUR JOURNEY

As a child, I had no idea that I would one day be stepping into my life's purpose of being my brother's caregiver. My brother's disability was not clear to me then, but I knew he was not like me, and knew that nor was he a normal kid. Autism, cerebral palsy, and scoliosis are my brother's diagnoses, coupled with being non-verbal. It is quite difficult when your loved one cannot express to you through words or signals how he feels, or how sick he is, but my bond with my brother is so strong that I can almost always tell when something is not right with him.

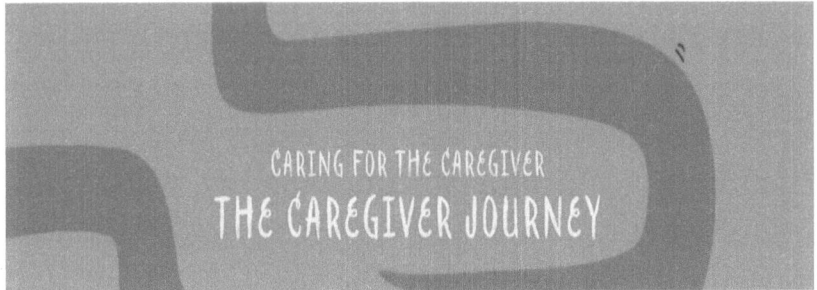

This is a story about the full-time job of caring for a sibling with a disability - despite the odds.

We were born in Washington, D.C., while our parents were still in college. Like most parents in my neighborhood, mine worked menial jobs to make ends meet. While they were at work, my brother and I were dropped off at the babysitter's or at a family friend's home.

I have memories of being scared and somewhat embarrassed to get on the bus with my mom and brother every morning, because he would scream, yell, and cry. We would get looks from passengers the entire bus ride. It was all part of his disability. This daily ordeal made me sad, and I couldn't hide it. I was unhappy, not because of the embarrassing tantrums, but because I wanted my brother to be a normal kid.

At two years old, Rolly still had difficulties learning how to walk, and he hadn't uttered a word. So, mom enrolled him in a school specifically for kids with disabilities. In no time, we started seeing improvements. I remember the joy I felt the first day I heard him speak. His exact words were, "thank you," "mommy," and "daddy." That day solidified the meaning of happiness for me. It was indeed a happy day for us all.

Before long, my dad withdrew my brother from the school and took both of us back to Nigeria. This happened unbeknownst to my mom, who'd had an aneurysm and was in the hospital fighting for her life. On the plane, I kept asking my dad where we were going, why we were on the plane, and where my mother was. When I didn't get the answers I wanted, I told one of the flight attendants that my dad was taking us back to Nigeria and that I did not want to go. The flight attendant asked if that was true, and my Dad (rest his soul) told her that we were going to see our grandparents and we would be back to the States soon. What I did not know at the time was that my grandparents on both my dad and mom's side were long gone, and that our "short visit" would turn into more than a decade. Dad had taken us back to Nigeria to attend law school and start up his law practice. It really took a village, literally, to take care of both of us, which is the norm in African families. Relatives, cousins, aunts, and uncles were all part of the journey.

CHAPTER 2: ENCOURAGEMENT

I honestly don't know where my courage comes from. The night before my friend helped me to bring my brother back from Nigeria, I had nightmares and was crying in my sleep, waking myself up. At that time, I knew that my life would completely change, that my freedom no longer existed, but I was okay with it, because I knew he needed me. I know that my courage and strength came from seeing him happy and being able to be a part of helping another human being live a full and deserving life.

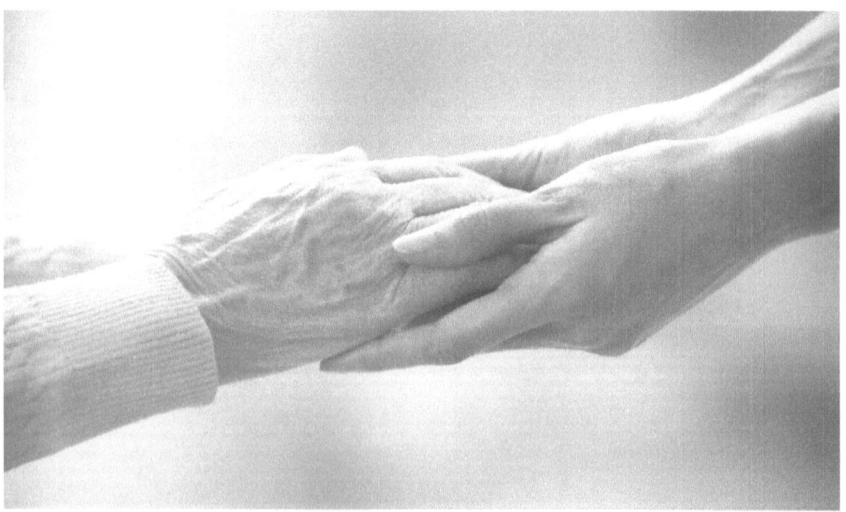

Most of the difficulties I encountered in the beginning stages were not knowing where to go for help, where to seek assistance, and sometimes, in finding the motivation to keep going.

Since my brother had been away from the United States for quite some time, I had to fill out a mountain of paperwork to access his services from the state. There was a waiting period for things to get approved. During that time, I had to figure out a way to make ends meet. Having a full-time job and going to school while being a caregiver was no small feat. At that time, it wasn't so easy to find the information I needed online. Finding out about resources available to me meant going to the Health and Human Services office, asking a lot of questions, and being persistent, which is exactly what I did. In some cases, you as a caregiver and your care recipient may not be eligible for nor qualify for some things. For instance, to qualify for a certain program could mean that the care recipient must be within a certain age range. When I first brought my brother back to the US, he didn't qualify for most support services because he was already 21, which the system typically considers as adult. This was especially difficult, and it meant I had to search for alternative ways to get him the help he needed. To this day, there are still a few things that he doesn't qualify for, such as sign language therapy/coaching. To pay for this service is quite a lot of money, which I can't afford at this time. So, if an organization cannot help you because you do not meet the criteria needed to be eligible for aid, you can always research, and make sure you ask questions about organizations that can provide assistance for your loved one.

I had no prior preparations, nor did I take a class in "caregiving" (I'm not sure such a class exists). In my case, something I can't explain activated my caregiving instincts. Granted, some people would not have similarly stepped up, family or not, but I love my brother so much that I didn't want to see him go without love and care. Also, since he is non-verbal, I have always felt the need to protect and look out for him.

Being a caregiver is not a learned skill. It comes naturally, and you learn a lot along the way. This role to me means more than simply giving care. It gives me joy to see my brother happy, getting the medical services he needs, and being able to live a full life. Are there times I feel overwhelmed and want to give up? Of course, but with a lot of perseverance and prayers, I've been able to pull through.

As much as being a sibling caregiver has been rewarding, it has also been challenging. Addressing the issue of being a sibling caregiver is very important, especially within different family dynamics. This provides the opportunity to discuss with family who would take over certain roles if anything unexpected were to happen. In my family, the caregiver issue was never discussed, so taking care of my brother is a role I didn't have to assume. I did it anyway, because no one else was stepping up. So, it is advisable to address caregiver roles in such a way that the burden doesn't fall on one person alone.

However, if you do find yourself in a solo caregiving role, please remember to take a break, as this is very essential. When you do not take a break, your stress will turn into frustration and exhaustion. The last thing you want to do is take out your anger on the person you are taking care of. As a caregiver, please take time to yourself and ask for help when you cannot keep up anymore. There are people out there willing to help.

Most disabilities or special needs challenges can also be a challenge for the caregiver, too, including major tantrums and emotional issues, many of which are never outgrown. For instance, when my brother was growing up, one of his tantrums involved breaking his plate when he wanted more food. Being non-verbal didn't help at all. It took the family a while to understand what was going on, but this is an example of a challenge we had to deal with by gradually showing him how to better communicate to ask for more food.

It is difficult to have a full work and school life all while having your own family and being a caregiver to a family member. My young adulthood was pretty much non-existent, but I had to find a way to make it work. Luckily, I had friends, neighbors, and family that were always willing to help, such as by "babysitting" for a few hours while I went out.

Although I had all this help, I still felt a little bit of guilt (It comes with the territory, but don't let it stop you). At the time, I was in college and working a full-time job. My work schedule was the 5am shift at a hardware store, and I took my break around 8am. During my break, I would rush home to give my brother breakfast, then rush back to work for another 4hrs, which got me home for lunch. Several times when I came home, the house was flooded because my brother would turn on the faucet and wouldn't know how to turn it back off.

Why would I would even think of leaving him alone? I am not proud of the fact that there were times I had to leave him by himself, but the short and simple answer is that I had to put food on the table and a roof over our heads. That same year, I dropped out of school for a semester because the pressure of so many competing demands had taken a toll on me. But I am here today, grateful to God that we got through that phase of our life, and YOU can and will too. My intention is to help make the journey easier for all Sibling Caregivers.

One thing I wish I did differently was to join a support group of "caregivers." But at the beginning stages of being a sibling caregiver, I was so busy trying to make ends meet that joining a support group was the farthest thing from my mind. Plus, I was a lot younger then, so I felt I had a handle on things. Even Super Woman needs a break sometimes, and things would have been a lot easier if I'd had a support group. Find a support group in your area. If there is none, then start one. You don't have to go on this journey alone. As much as your family needs you to take care of them, you need other people to lean on, too.

CHAPTER 3: WHO IS A SIBLING CAREGIVER?

Informal caregivers are family members, friends, or neighbors who help to provide care for an individual suffering from an acute or chronic condition who needs help to cope with day-to-day activities. Informal caregivers are usually actively involved in the caretaking responsibilities of a weak or disabled person. The work of informal caregivers all over the world is highly underappreciated, as they do more than just watch, feed, and help disabled people move around; they also have to listen all day to the care recipient, look out closely for any signs of an illness (as sufferers may not be able to communicate their discomfort properly), offer constant warmth and companionship, and in more cases than not, offer emotional support to their care recipients to help them alleviate anxiety and promote their general well-being.

According to the New York Consolidated Law Service, "An informal caregiver shall mean a family member or any other natural person who normally provides the daily care or supervision of a frail or disabled person, or any family member or other natural person who contributes to, and is involved in the caretaking responsibilities for such frail or disabled person. Such informal caregiver may, but need not, reside in the same household as the frail or disabled person."

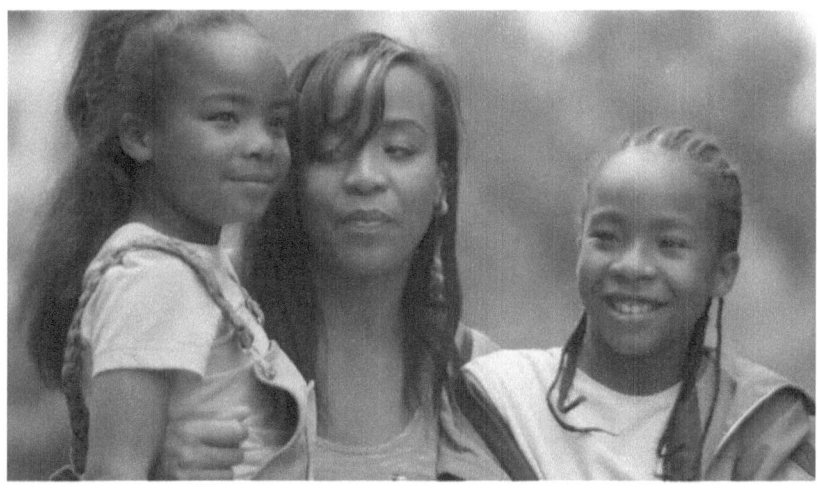

Sibling caregivers are siblings of physically challenged people who help to care for the physical and emotional needs of their disabled family member. In the case of sibling caregivers, it is common to find the siblings living together in the same house, with the sibling providing full-time support for the challenged family member, especially in cases where the disability is quite advanced and the disabled would find it difficult to cope alone without constantly having someone nearby. Siblings have the potential to be excellent caregivers, because they know the person they are caring for. Most older siblings start caring for their younger family members with special needs when they are still young, assisting their parents and offering constant emotional support to their sibling every day. As normal siblings grow up, a special type of bond usually forms, a bond borne of growing up together, going through great and challenging times together, celebrating successes and consoling each other in times of failure. Research has shown that this bond is usually stronger between a normal sibling and an autistic sibling or sibling with special needs. This is because as normal siblings grow up, they become individually independent. Most times, during the teenage years, adolescents tend to get closer to their friends, and their bonds with their siblings may not be as strong as before, as they are now relatively independent, both emotionally and physically. As regular adolescents reach their mid-teenage years, they begin to spend more time with their friends or love interests, and by adulthood, that strong bond that was formed in childhood may not be so strong anymore.

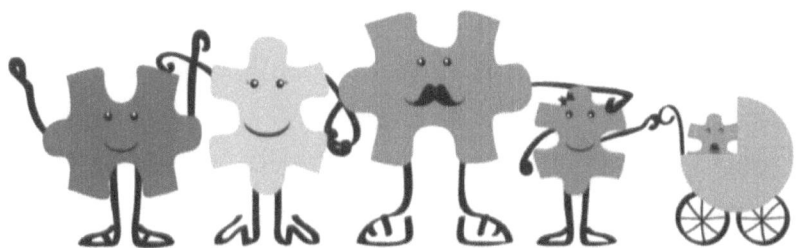

The Whole Autism Family

Autistic Spectrum Disorder (ASD) is a developmental disability characterized by difficulties in social interaction, communication and by restricted or repetitve patterns of thought and behavior.

In examining the relationship between siblings and autistic family members, however, it is noticed that the autistic family member would normally need the support of his/her family to cope with his/her day-to-day life. Most challenged people usually find it more difficult, relatively, to make friends, especially children suffering from autism. Therefore, they tend to relate almost exclusively with their siblings and parents during childhood. While regular teenagers would usually make a lot of friends during their teenage years and slowly drift away from their families, autistic teenagers grow even closer to their siblings during adolescence. Even if the autistic child goes to a special school where he can make friends with other challenged kids, he may not be able to effectively take care of himself while at home. This will necessitate the assistance of a sibling caregiver, who will tend to his daily care, and transport him to and from school and other activities. If a single sibling cares for a challenged family member more than any other member of the family for a long time, an incomparable bond forms. The sibling caregiver will know almost everything about their sibling with special needs. This would make caring for their sibling an integral part of their daily life, and not just a job as an external caregiver would see it.

Growing up with my brother, he and I certainly formed a bond that most people can't seem to understand. Although he is non-verbal, I can tell when he doesn't feel well, when he's upset, or when something is bothering him. All of this became the norm because we lived in the same household growing up.

Therefore, a sibling who grew up caring for an autistic family member is one of the best caregivers that a sibling with special needs can have. In most cases, the solid emotional bond that has been built through childhood and adolescence continues to get stronger with every passing day, as the sibling caregiver will usually find satisfaction and fulfillment in helping to keep his autistic sibling well and happy. As fulfilling and honorable as being a sibling caregiver can be, it also comes with many challenges.

Life can sometimes get busy with daily schedules, and some days are harder to manage than others. There are goals to be achieved, deadlines to meet, and more, coupled with other personal challenges. Caring for a sibling with a disability every day, while still trying to keep your personal life in order, may just be one of the most tedious and exhausting lifestyles in the world. Virtually all sibling caregivers had life goals and objectives prior to stepping into the role of caregiver, but the fact that most people cannot bear to abandon their siblings with special needs in a bid to pursue their own personal objectives means that they might have to make some important sacrifices. These in turn could affect and sometimes pause their careers and other life goals.

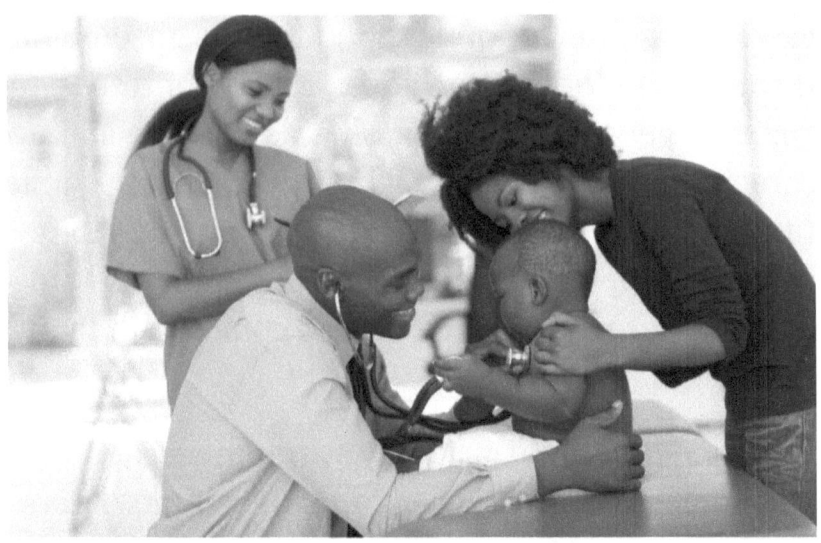

One of the most important challenges sibling caregivers must face is being forced to limit the scope of the activities they can engage in, just to see to the well-being of their sibling with special needs. Personally, I had to not only adjust my work and school schedule to take care of my brother, but as a young adult at the time, I had to pass up on doing things with friends, traveling, and study abroad opportunities. One of the biggest decisions I made was to step into the caregiver role for my brother, but I wouldn't have it any other way. At the beginning of our sibling caregiver journey, a lot of times, I was torn between chasing my dreams and caring for my brother. But each time I came to the conclusion that being his caregiver was one of my purposes here on Earth. While different caregivers usually make varying decisions when faced with puzzling situations, in which they have to choose between family and themselves, it definitely takes a strong person to deny him/herself an opportunity because of their love for a family member.

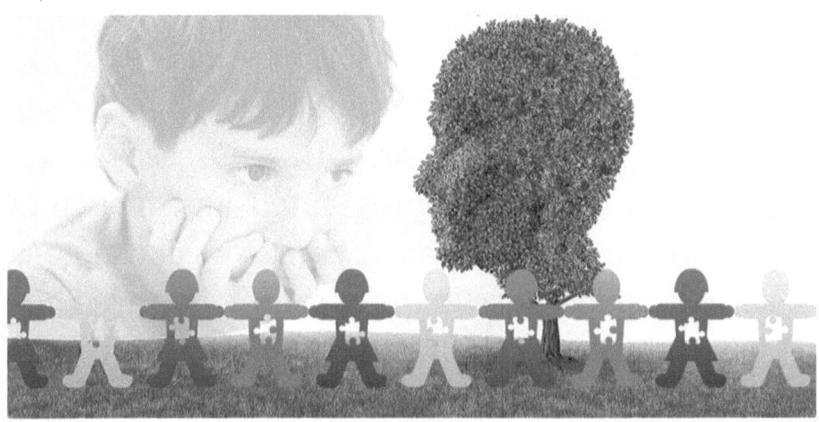

To help ease the strain that being a caregiver can have on one's personal life, and to help make the achievement of one's personal goals easier, one can enroll a sibling with special needs in a community living environment, specifically meant for people with his or her kind of disability. This can be an efficient way to help with your caregiver journey. However, it requires you having trust in the people you've placed your loved one with. Before choosing a community living home for your loved one, however, it is important to do your research and run adequate background checks on the institution to confirm the dedication and experience of their caregivers and the suitability of the environment for the needs of your loved one. In a lot of cases, caregivers in special care centers (and sometimes caregivers hired to care for a loved one at home) have been reported to viciously abuse the patients they were meant to take care of, both physically and emotionally. In a painful video that went viral a few years ago, a caregiver was seen mercilessly hitting an autistic patient, probably out of frustration, over and over until the patient bled. In some cases, some of these caregivers get prosecuted and justice is served, but in a lot of cases, caregiver abuse goes unaddressed, because many of the victims are non-verbal and cannot appropriately express the pain they are going through at the hands of those who are supposed to be helping make their dark days a little brighter.

Another very common difficulty that sibling caregivers face in the discharge of their duties is intense physical stress. Combining school, work, and maintaining an active social life is exhausting as it is. Coupled with the duties of being a caregiver every day, the stress only compounds. In a lot of cases, sibling caregivers have been reported to come down with severe cases of exhaustion, and in some extreme cases, conditions like high blood pressure and hypertension. While it is important to properly care for a challenged loved one to ensure that they do not inadvertently hurt themselves or others, it is also very essential to keep your personal life as a caregiver in check. Therefore, although striking a balance between your personal life and your duties as a caregiver may be intensely exhausting, it is also important for you to find time to rest, to ensure your personal well-being and the well-being of your loved one with special needs. To help relieve the physical stress that comes with your duties, you can ask for the help of other family members, friends, or neighbors who you think can be of assistance while you get some well-deserved rest. Coming down with bouts of depression won't do you or your care recipient any good.

Due to the intense stress that the job of a caregiver entails, combining being a caregiver with running an active personal life can also cause severe emotional stress. Research indicates that 75% of informal caregivers have complained of the high emotional stress attached to their job. 60% of informal caregivers said being a caregiver had made their health significantly worse. Emotional stress stemming from caregiving work may be caused by a number of things. One factor that can cause great emotional stress is the stigma and isolation that a lot of sibling caregivers all over the world are faced with while caring for their loved ones. As a young child, I used to feel quite embarrassed and hurt by the long, weird stares that I and my brother received from people any time we were out in public. This stigma and isolation can lead to severe emotional stress, especially if the autistic/special needs family member throws occasional tantrums in public. While members of society who stigmatize people with special needs and their caregivers need to work on their attitudes, sibling caregivers may benefit from counseling sessions which involve fellow informal caregivers and experienced mental health professionals to help ease severe emotional stress.

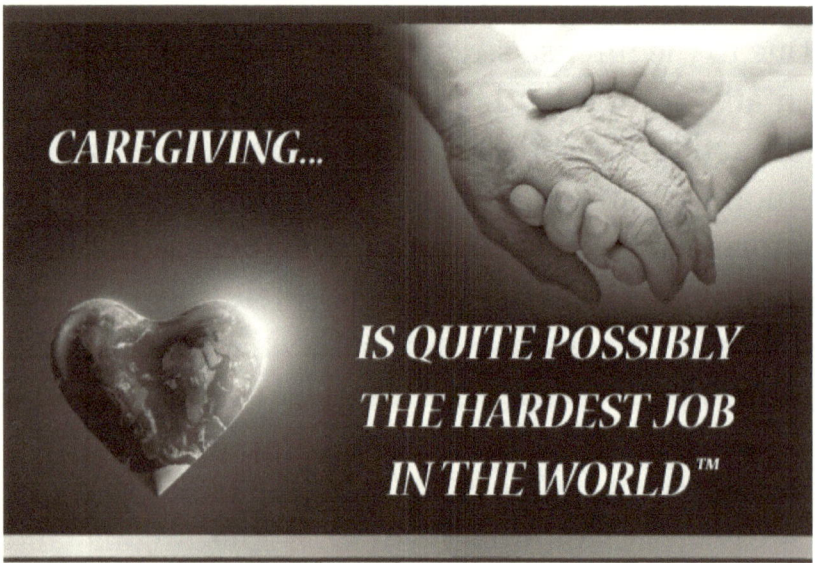

Another difficulty that many sibling caregivers face while caring for their challenged care recipient pertains to finding appropriate support services for their challenged care recipients in their local community. In a lot of areas, especially in the countryside, they do not have sufficient support structures to cater to the challenged population. When a caregiver cannot find support services, such as adult day care centers and government social care centers, for his care recipient, serious difficulties may arise that can disturb the personal life of the caregiver or hamper the quality of care that the care recipient has access to. Other services, like peer support and case management, are almost non-existent in many communities in the country.

Some of the difficulties that I faced personally being a sibling caregiver were the day-to-day tasks, exhaustion, and the motivation to set and accomplish my personal goals. For the most part, I have been my brother's primary caregiver for the past seventeen years. However, community living homes and adult day care centers (which will be talked about in subsequent chapters) have helped make the process a lot easier. Most of the difficulties I faced in the beginning were a result of not knowing where to go for help, when to seek assistance, or how to go about getting my brother back into the swing of things since we'd been away from the United States for so long. At that time, information wasn't as readily available as it is today.

However, I was able to pull through by constantly visiting the county social services office and asking a lot of questions. Even though there was still a waiting period for a few things to get finalized and approved for him, seeking help from the right places made things a lot easier for us. During the waiting period, I managed to find alternative means to making ends meet while at work and school, and of course while caring for my brother.

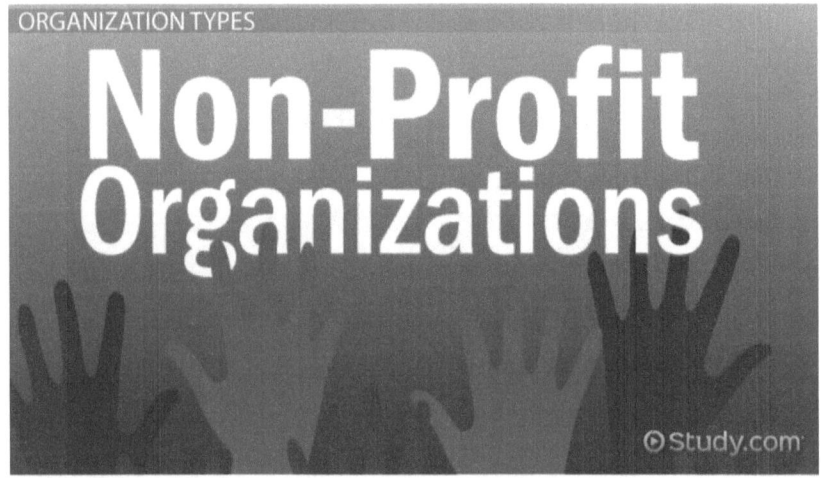

To help make the work of dedicated caregivers easier, the government and non-profit organizations, or, as they are known in some countries, non-governmental organizations (NGOs), need to help put some of these social care facilities in place in regions that are seriously in need. Imagine needing to travel from Texas to New Jersey for a very important job interview for three days. Even if you can afford to bring your sibling along to New Jersey due to the absence of social care facilities in your area in Texas, would you take your sibling with special needs along to your job interview in New Jersey? No. Therefore, while sibling caregivers may love their siblings with special needs unconditionally, there are always going to be situations in which the sibling caregiver must enlist the service of quality, informal caregiving professionals to help take care of their sibling while they attend to other pressing matters for extended periods of time. Easily accessible care should be made available for people with special needs without having to deal with so much red tape.

In addition, one of the most pressing challenges that sibling caregivers and their care recipients have to face today is the challenge of inadequate healthcare services. While there may be hospitals and clinics on every corner, dedicated healthcare centers catering to the needs of autistic patients still remain in short supply due to the fact that autism is still not fully understood by many. Services such as in-patient treatment and treatment for substance abuse need to be incorporated into the scope of local healthcare centers and dedicated care centers for individuals with special needs. While an untrained sibling caregiver may be able to offer physical and emotional support to the best of his/her ability, if he hasn't been trained as a medical expert, there will be little he/she can do in the case of a medical emergency. To help facilitate improved healthcare for autistic patients, the state, with the help of non-profit organizations, needs to invest in the provision of appropriate healthcare facilities and incorporate essential medical services into the scope of existing care centers. This will not only improve the quality of health of the autistic population, but will also help ease the stress that informal caregivers are forced to deal with in cases of medical emergencies.

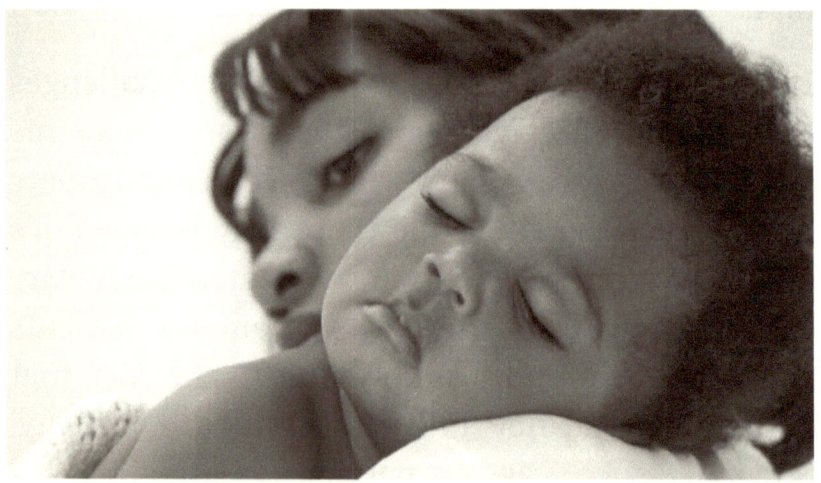

A different sort of issue that many sibling caregivers must grapple with is the issue of financial constraint. Taking care of a special needs family member is not an easy task physically, emotionally, or financially. In cases where the sibling caregiver must also financially provide for the needs of the care recipient, things can become quite difficult, especially if the sibling caregiver is not receiving any financial assistance for their duties as a caregiver. In severe cases of physical disability where the care recipient needs to use expensive medical equipment on a regular basis, financial difficulties compound even further, especially if the sibling caregiver does not have a well-paying job. Thankfully, major steps have been taken by the government to help relieve the financial stress that sibling caregivers face. Depending on the disability the care recipient has, he or she may be entitled to a periodic social security disbursement. Sibling caregivers who take care of their siblings with a disability full-time are entitled to get paid through the Medicaid program. Health insurance can also help cover some extensive medical costs. All in all, to avoid intense financial difficulty, sibling caregivers are encouraged to explore all available avenues to help ensure financial security for themselves and their care recipients. To get information about financial assistance available to people with a disability, or to care recipients of a particular age range, all feasible avenues, including social services, healthcare centers, and even the internet should be utilized. Ensuring access to all available funds to help lessen financial stress should be the aim. The value of unpaid informal caregiver work in the United States has reached about $257 billion per year. This is a huge amount, and informal caregivers really should reach out, gather information, and ensure they are paid and also get appropriate financial assistance for their care recipient. Paid professional caregivers in the United States can earn as much as $17 to $49 per hour. While this may be expensive for you as a sibling caregiver, you should consider temporarily hiring a private caregiver for your sibling with a disability. This gives insight to unpaid family caregivers about how valuable their services are, convincing most to accept financial assistance regardless of any cultural or ethnic beliefs stating otherwise.

Lack of access to useful information is a huge challenge that many caregivers have been facing for a very long time, and which they still have to grapple with today. The information needed to successfully care for a challenged care recipient can come in different forms. Medical-related information is perhaps the most important that a caregiver should have at hand while caring for a care recipient, especially one with a serious disability that can lead to violent or destructive behaviors. Caregivers should be adequately equipped with information related to medical emergencies through first-aid training such as CPR for cases of sudden violent attacks or loss of consciousness. Regular first-aid equipment should also be on hand in case the care recipient gets injured. The caregiver should be familiar with simple first-aid procedures, and important information like emergency hotline numbers and other essential contacts should be available in case the care recipient accidentally starts a fire or injures himself.

Apart from medical information, a caregiver should try as much as possible to get to know the care recipient. Things like the recipient's likes and dislikes and allergies should be known to the caregiver. The recipient's tolerance levels for disturbances such as noise, crowds, and stress should also be known to the caregiver, as these sorts of things differ among patients, and autistic patients tend to be more sensitive to things like stress and noise than those not on the spectrum. Luckily, access to information has been greatly improved in the modern world. With the advent of the internet, caregivers all over the world can now access information relating to the mannerisms or the challenges their care recipients suffer from, applicable first-aid procedures, and things to avoid when taking care of a special-needs person. With the help of the internet, too, opportunities for financial assistance for both the caregiver and the care recipient are now easily accessible. This can go a long way in lessening the burden on a family caregiver and improve the quality of life and health of the healthcare recipient. In cases where the internet is not of much help in accessing information on how to deal with a specific issue your loved one or care recipient may be dealing with, contact your local social services or an experienced healthcare professional to help. Knowledge is power, after all.

When dealing with your county social services or social security office for any kind of assistance, keep in mind that the process does take a while, so be patient. It may take quite some time for the center to respond to your complaint or inquiry. During this waiting period, you may have to deal with financial challenges and technical difficulties, such as the lack of a ventilator, wheelchair, or respite services for a care recipient, all of which could alleviate you of some of your day-to-day activities. During this waiting period, a caregiver may have to ask for financial and physical support from other family members and friends. Also, while waiting to hear back from social services, it is important to start researching a community living home for your loved one, if that is the direction you decide to go. A primary care physician will also be critical to your loved one's progress.

The purpose of this book is to let sibling caregivers, and all caregivers, know that they are not alone in their journey. Answering the questions below is the first step.

    A. When did you find out that you were taking over the duties of being a caregiver?

    B. Did you know that you needed training to be a caregiver? If not, how have you been able to manage on your own?

    C. What did you expect stepping into this role as a caregiver?

CHAPTER 4: ACCEPTANCE

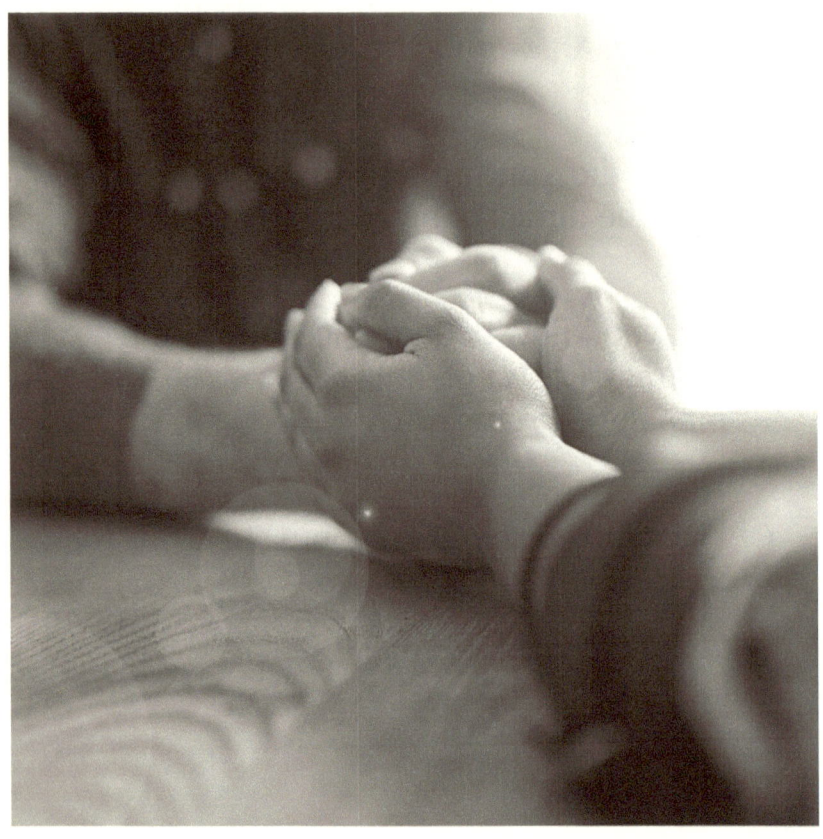

Acceptance begins from within. Being in the role of a sibling caregiver may be hard to accept at first, but the earlier you do, the better. It is important to realize that taking care of your loved one is now your new normal. In my situation, I had to get to a point where I could accept that my brother and I were stuck with each other, so to speak. I had to let other people in my life (present and future) know that my brother was, is, and will always be a huge part of my life.

As a young adult, it was difficult having to stay at home while my friends went out partying, took vacations, met new people, and made new friends. Plenty of times, I questioned why I had taken on the role of sibling caregiver. There were a lot of times I wanted to give up. But believe it or not, next to having your own kids, being a caregiver is one of the most rewarding experiences you can have. You'll learn so much about yourself and your sibling. If your sibling is non-verbal, like mine, the level of interaction both of you can have will be beyond understanding both to you and to others who watch and see what an amazing job you are doing! It always helps to put things in perspective, first by looking within and finding that place of gratitude and love, then by drawing from your inner strength and achieving acceptance.

I don't blame or point fingers at anyone for putting me in this role. With all the different family dynamics out there, some loose ends have to get picked up by someone. Of course, I have my days when I get frustrated and tired, but God has given me the strength to carry out this mission. This is something you will have to live with for a long time, even if you place your loved one in a group home or community living center. If you are not at a place where you have fully accepted your role as caregiver, it will certainly show, and you might take it out on the person you are caring for.

Some family caregivers find their role as a caregiver challenging and tedious. They sometimes dislike being a caregiver, and rightfully so. This doesn't mean these people are bad or that caregiving is a terrible thing to do, but the truth is, when you haven't learned to accept a situation, you will never be able to view it quite objectively. While being a caregiver is very rewarding and fulfilling, the love for the person you are caring for must stem from the deepest part of your heart. You must love them with no holds barred. You must be willing to help them grow and develop. The point is, a forced caregiver will probably end up as a bad caregiver.

When people hate their jobs, it's only natural that they will always find a fault with their work. When you hate caregiving as a responsibility, or when you haven't allowed yourself to come to terms with the fact that you are now a caregiver, you really shouldn't assume the role of being one yet; at least, not fully. It is when you learn to accept the situation on its face, when you manage to come to terms with the fact that you now toned to dedicate your energy, time, attention, and, most of all, love to a person with special needs who would find it difficult to survive without your help, it is then that you are ready to become a caregiver. The amazing thing about learning to accept harsh realities is that, as soon as you come to terms with the situation, coping with the challenges that come with that responsibility becomes progressively easier. You won't see fixing meals, doing laundry, and pushing the person around on a wheelchair as challenging. You will begin to see your responsibilities, and yourself, in a new light. When you learn to accept the role of caregiver wholeheartedly, then you are ready to help your care recipient embark on the journey ahead.

There are a number of factors that can make accepting the caregiver role difficult, even before you assume the responsibilities associated with such acceptance. One of the major factors that usually deters caregivers, especially young family caregivers, from accepting their roles as sibling caregivers is, "*WHAT WOULD PEOPLE SAY?*" The harsh reality of the world we live in today is that a lot of people now care more about other people's opinions than they do about that actually matter. Personally, I have a mantra I abide by that has made me stand strong even when the emotional stress of caregiving becomes almost unbearable.

The mantra is, "The people who care don't matter and the people who matter don't care." As cliché as it might be, there is a lot of truth to it. As soon as you learn to live by this "cliché," your problems become easier to solve. In life generally, people always worry about what people think about them, and in the process, they lose focus on what is supposed to be done. As a caregiver, you need to understand that whatever you do, people will talk. If a young, ambitious, and hardworking young adult buys a nice car, people might say that he/she could be drug dealing or defrauding people. If that same young adult uses public transportation to get around, those same people will still have something negative to say. The point is: stop allowing society to dictate your life. Learn to have strong decision-making skills, learn to speak your truth, and face adversity head-on, no matter what life throws at you.

Yes. The world is a very complicated place, and we do not always get what we deserve, at times. But when you learn to realize that life is not fair, you learn to be firm and strong and take on every challenge that life throws at you. If you need to talk to someone, please do, but before you embark on this tedious but rewarding journey as a caregiver, you need to carefully weigh your options and strengthen your mind. You need to get yourself ready emotionally to cope with the emotional stress and discouragements that will come your way as you take on your duties as a caregiver. When you learn to make your own decisions without worrying about what other people might say, accepting your role as a caregiver will become so much easier.

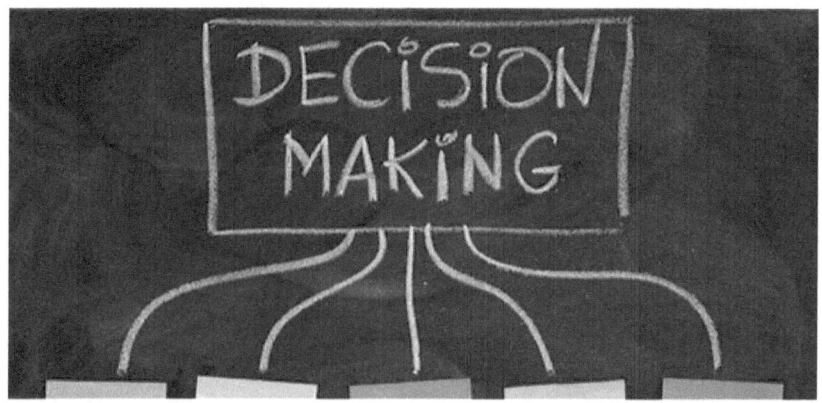

Another salient factor that makes accepting a caregiving role quite difficult is the consideration of how you will manage to juggle other aspects of your life, such as school or work, with the naturally tedious job of caring for a loved one with special needs. Before you jump into this role truthfully, you really need to look critically at your current engagements. How much work can you delegate elsewhere to free up more time to care for your care recipient? Would there be any form of help or assistance from friends and family when things get challenging? You must look objectively at your current schedule to see how well you can manage caregiving roles and other duties to ensure there are minimal glitches on both sides. After carefully evaluating your schedules and deciding how you can create time to care for your loved one as much as possible, you can then talk to friends and family, preferably close, long-term friends and immediate family members who actually know the care recipient to some extent. After you have found a way to carefully plan out your time to include ample and reasonable periods of caregiving, work or school, and rest, you can be assured that you won't have to worry about your care recipient while at work, and neither should you have to worry too much about work while caring for your love.

Sometimes, planning how to effectively be a caregiver is not always possible. In my case, I tried to plan, but in the end, I learned to be a caregiver while on the job. However, my reason for writing this book was so that readers would be able to learn from my journey and apply my insights to their caregiver journeys accordingly. So, if after carefully evaluating your schedule, you find that there just doesn't seem to be enough time to fit in caregiving duties, you may have to make a very crucial decision. Are you willing to sacrifice a part of your personal life for the sake of another person? It is very important not to rush into caregiving duties, or else issues like caregiver abuse and depression can come up when you eventually begin. Therefore, before starting out as a caregiver, it is important to come to terms with the situation you are faced with, to understand how being a caregiver will change the life you used to have. It is also important to consult the right people, who can help when things get quite challenging, and finally, it is important to make the needed sacrifices once and for all. Let your job know what your situation is from the time you get hired, or whenever you assume your caregiver duties. Doing so will put you and your supervisor in a place of understanding should emergencies arise. Often, I had to leave work or school early to attend to issues that pertained to my brother, and my supervisors or teachers were always quite understanding. The sooner you make your decisions and get around to implementing your plans, the easier it will be to accept your new role as a caregiver and the easier it will be to cope with the challenges that comes with doing one of the most honorable and rewarding jobs in the world: caring for a loved one in need.

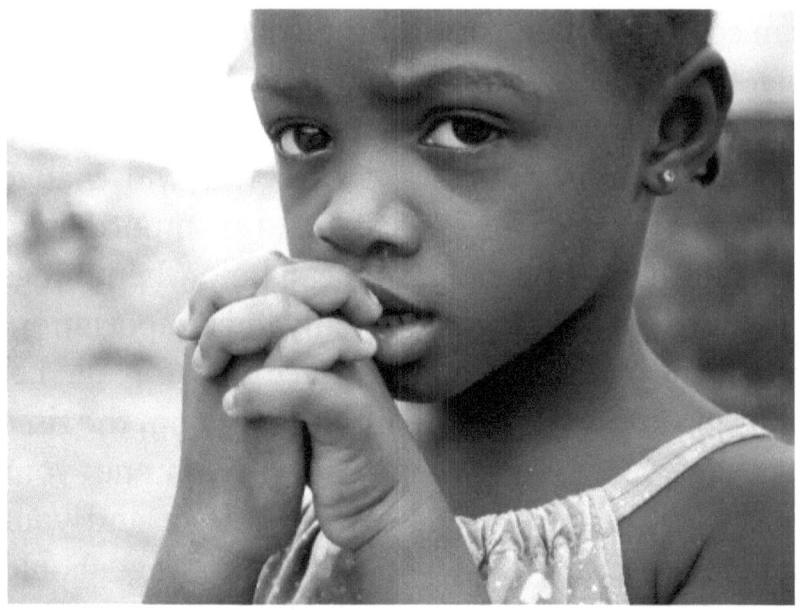

Another factor that makes it difficult for most young adults to accept the role of caregiver is the fear that their social lives will suffer. To be honest, being a good caregiver can deprive you of some of the luxuries you may be used to. You might not be as free to attend Friday night parties anymore, and you may not be able to hang out with your friends from school or your colleagues from work every weekend, either. Just because you will need to care for your disabled care recipient, you may have to decline a request from someone dear to you and in some cases you will not be able to help your friends out when they need you. Personally, I had to give up quite a chunk of my young adult life. However, I still found ways to incorporate fun into my life as much as I could. I began to realize that the friends who really didn't know much about my caregiver duties gradually became distant, and they probably looked at me as a party pooper. I did lose some good friends in the process. The point is, don't be ashamed to tell people in your life about your new caregiving role. You'd be surprised at how understanding and supportive they will often be.

Let your friends help you accept your new job being a caregiver to your loved one. Their support and encouragement are all you need sometimes. Also, having a family member or a neighbor help out from time to time frees you up to hang out and spend time with your friends.

Accepting your role as a caregiver will give you the strength and determination you'll need to forge ahead and perform outstandingly in your caregiving work, even if you are not getting paid for it. Most caregivers are usually concerned however, about how they will cope, how they will manage to properly function in a capacity that they have not been trained to serve in. The anxiety and worry that a lot of people experience as to how they will care for someone entirely on their own is one of the factors that makes acceptance difficult for most prospective caregivers.

While it is true that lack of proper training in how to carry out duties specific to being a caregiver can hamper a caregiver's ability to properly care for a person with special needs, it is also true that most of the fears people entertain before starting out on any endeavor, caregiving inclusive, are totally unfounded. A considerable percentage of caregivers all over the world have not undergone any kind of special training to make them better-suited to carry out caregiving duties. A majority of these untrained caregivers are still managing to care properly, if not perfectly, for their loved ones in need. Learning to be a good caregiver is not solely about getting special training. Caregiving, more than anything else, is about loving and being concerned for the welfare of a person. When you can find it in your heart to care truly for a loved one in need, to love them, not just because you pity them but because you are passionate about seeing them grow and thrive, you indeed have what it takes to be a fantastic caregiver! The fact that you truly love and care about your care recipient does not mean those jeers on the street won't hurt, but if you have accepted to care for this person whom you love so much it will make it easier and more comfortable to do so in peace.

Therefore, to make accepting the situation a reality and fitting into the role of an informal caregiver easier, it is important to realize that all you need is love. You can attend caregiving training seminars, research information on how to be a great caregiver online, or take a medical course just to help care for your loved one with special needs, but if you are not truly concerned about the welfare of the person you will be taking care of, then being a caregiver will become progressively more difficult. To make acceptance easier, I want you to understand that although being trained as a caregiver might be important, especially for care recipients with serious disorders, the most important thing to possess before setting out to care for a person with special needs is a genuine concern for that person's wellbeing. Love conquers all, as they say. If you are anxious about stepping into the role because your care recipient has a chronic disorder, or because you just can't summon the courage to step into it without some prior training, there are several avenues available to you which you can use to receive some training and assistance regarding how to be a better caregiver. If you are anxious about how you'd cope with the financial-related duties associated with being a caregiver, several organizations exist to help you. In the next chapters, I'll detail the resources available to help you in your caregiving journey.

One other thing that calls for concern, which usually bothers most soon-to-be caregivers, is how they will adapt to the new way of life that caregiving introduces them to and how to manage taking care of oneself in the process. It is normal to feel somewhat jittery about adjusting to this new, intimidating way of life that caregiving will thrust you into. It could be more difficult for outgoing people and extroverts to switch from hanging out with friends and attending meetings to staying in all day with someone who may not even be able to keep up with regular conversation. Apart from having to cope with staying all alone with a care recipient, new caregivers may also have to learn new skills and inculcate new habits. Knowledge related to medical terminologies, managing complex finances, and finding legal representation for they and their loved ones are just a few of the tricky issues that new caregivers will have to cope with.

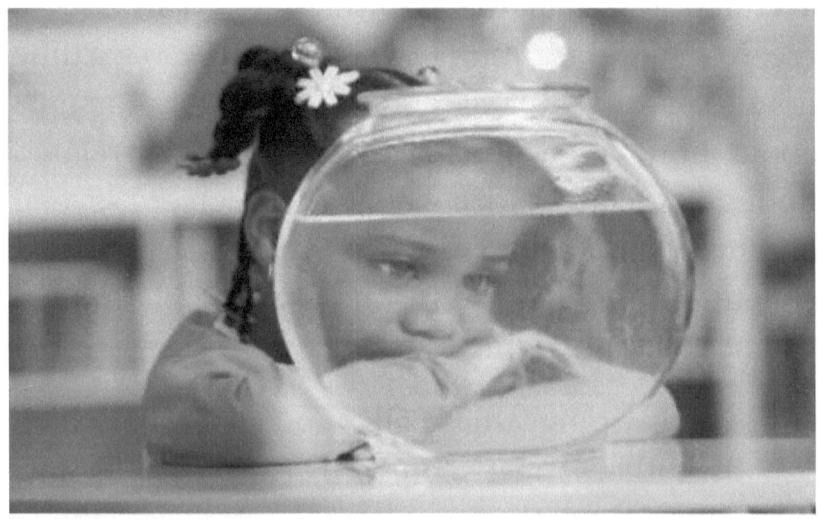

Personally, I believe it's okay to have these kinds of fears when stepping into a new role as a caregiver. What I do not believe is that it is acceptable to allow these fears to stop you from doing what's right. The human brain is quite complex and has an almost infinite capacity to store information. As time goes on, you will learn to be proficient in everything that has ever scared you about caregiving. Proper planning and help from friends and family can also help allay your fears about adjusting to this new pattern of life and still finding time to take care of yourself. Once you truly care about the well-being of the person you are caring for, the courage and eagerness to learn and practice what you learn, the strength to do everything you need to do, and the opportunities to meet the right people who can provide help just come naturally.

In cases where for one reason or another, you simply cannot step into your caregiving role, there are various medically approved facilities that can help take care of your loved one with special needs while you tend to your personal life. It is, however, important to spend some amount of time, no matter how little, with your loved one, to show that you truly care about them, especially when they no longer live with you.

As a caregiver, it is important to avoid "caregiver burnout." If you are caring for a close family member, there should be someone who can relieve you of your duties for a day or two while you rest and hang out with friends. Getting enough rest and socializing with others is important for caregivers to prevent caregiver abuse. What is the use of your dedication as a caregiver when you end up taking out your anger and stress on your loved one? Knowing your personal stress threshold as a caregiver is very important. It's okay to push yourself to the limits in order to provide care to your care recipient to the best of your ability, but this must be done within reasonable limits.

It is very easy to be oblivious to how our daily activities wear us out physically and emotionally. When serving as a caregiver, however, you'll experience higher levels of emotional stress, which usually has a more devastating effect on the mind, making chronic emotional stress an almost automatic precursor to caregiver abuse. You may think there is nothing in the world that could drive you to abuse or assault your loved one, but when you are over the edge and emotionally stressed out, you can end up surprising yourself with your actions. It is very important, therefore, for every caregiver to find enough time to rest properly while carrying out their caregiving duties. Apart from caregiver abuse, there are other consequences that exhaustion and chronic physical and emotional stress can have on your health as a caregiver. Issues ranging from intense muscular pain and dizziness to depression, high blood pressure, and hypertension are issues of concern when it comes to the health of caregivers. Take time out to rest, for your own benefit, and for the benefit of your care recipient and everyone else around you.

In the caregiver world, it cannot be emphasized enough how important self-care and rest are. Here are a few questions you need to ask yourself to ensure that you are taking care of yourself:

A. On a scale of 1-10, with 10 being the highest, how stressful are your caregiver duties?

B. What about your caregiving makes it so stressful for you at the present moment? (This can all change)

How many days out of the week or month do you take a break from your caregiving responsibilities?

C. Do you have a friend or family member who can help you during emergencies? List all their names and numbers.

D. Do you have access to resources in your community that offer respite services? If so, list them. If not, research and come back to this page with what you found.

Prior to now, list areas you could improve upon when it comes to better self-care.

CHAPTER 5: THE CAREGIVERS' INCREDIBLE GIFTS, AND THE PEOPLE WHO DON'T APPRECIATE THEM

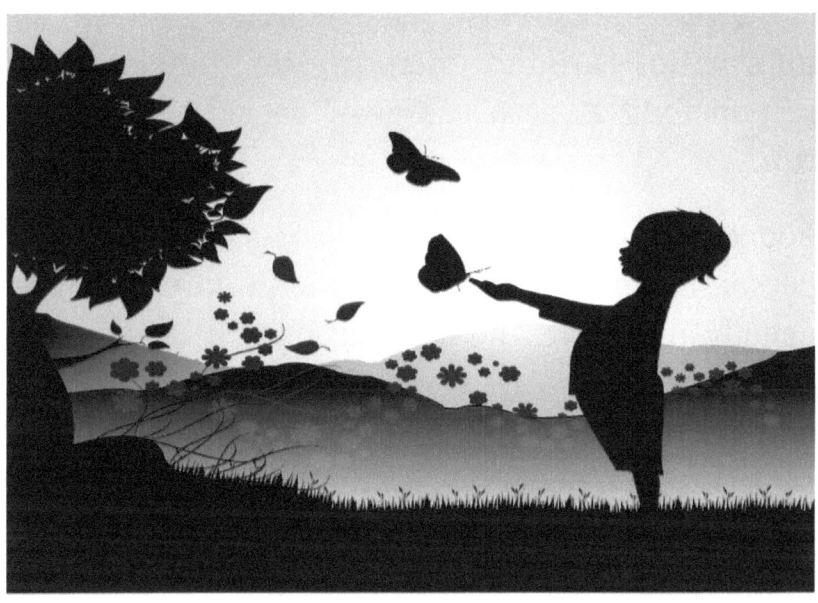

Often overlooked is the fact that sibling caregivers usually do not possess any sort of professional training regarding the work they do. Most paid professional caregivers have undergone professional training, and usually they have medical knowledge in case of emergencies. However, a sibling caregiver has to offer a lot more that cannot be learned – energy, time, and unconditional love. Therefore, being an untrained sibling caregiver is challenging enough, let alone having to combine lack of proper training with lack of resources to appropriately care for the care recipient. While it may not be possible for every informal caregiver all over the world to receive formal training on how to properly care for someone with special needs, it is advisable that caregivers make use of reliable sources of information around them to help make their responsibilities as a caregiver easier in the long run.

People who have had to care for a seriously sick person or an aged person at one point or another usually appreciate the role that informal caregivers play in society. Due to their lack of both training and prior experience, it is not uncommon to see such caregivers buckling under the intense strain of their responsibilities, especially in periods of crisis when extra attention must be paid to the care recipient. According to research, two categories of people usually underestimate and overlook the roles that caregivers play in society: people with absolutely no experience of being a caregiver and healthcare professionals who see no use in training informal caregivers. It is easy to understand why people who have never acted in any capacity as a caregiver for a sick or aged person might underestimate the work of caregivers. Experience, they say, is the best teacher, after all. Some people who have never cared for a person with special needs do not understand what such work entails. They often think the work of caregivers is minor, or unworthy of note. This is not the case, however. Apart from the physical stress that caregivers cope with as they attend to the numerous everyday needs of their recipients, the emotional toll that comes with caregiving is enormous. It is not unusual to hear of sibling caregivers coming down with mild to severe cases of depression, especially when their care recipients are suffering from a crisis or relapse of some sort. People who don't understand this line of work should learn to respect and assist caregivers when they can. Isolating and stigmatizing caregivers and their care recipients in public settings, corporate settings, and even in the neighborhood should be stopped. People need to learn to understand the rigors and stress that come with being someone's caregiver. The responsibility is enormous, and their work shouldn't ever go unappreciated.

Another category of people who may not appreciate the work of informal caregivers as much as they should are found in an unlikely place: some healthcare fields. Most doctors, nurses, interns, and even non-medical staff at hospitals greatly respect the work that family caregivers do, especially considering that these caregivers do not usually undergo formal training before being thrown into the tedious world of informal care. The fact that these healthcare professionals also play some caregiving roles in their duties to patients with special needs puts them in a position to, more than anybody else, understand and appreciate the work that caregivers do. However, some healthcare professionals do not see the need for informal caregivers to undergo any sort of training before performing their duties as caregivers to their care recipients. This category of healthcare professional believes that caring for a loved one with special needs is not a job that requires training, but one that requires love and compassion only. While love and compassion, in addition to some other requirements like dedication and hard work, are some of the qualities of a great caregiver, this does not negate the fact that caregivers who have undergone some sort of training, whether formal or informal, are likely to be able to care better for their care recipients than their totally untrained counterparts.

Sibling Caregiver

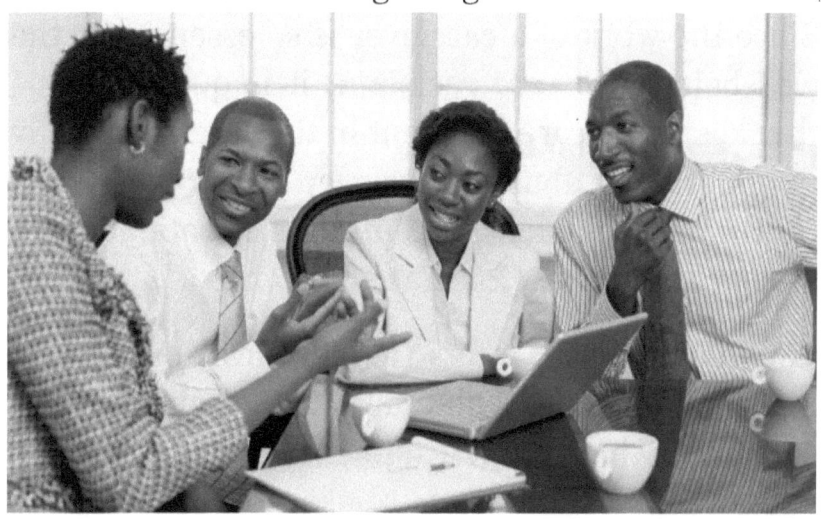

To this end, semi-formal training programs with practical sessions can be organized by non-profit organizations or healthcare professionals whose focus is on assisting caregivers. Such training could entail how to care properly for care recipients, steps to take in cases of emergencies, and how to specifically care for individuals with special needs. Periodically, organizations such as group homes, community living homes, and adult day care programs can distribute relief materials to people with special needs and their caregivers to help better cater to the individuals receiving care. Ultimately, it is important for organizations and agencies to effectively communicate and have best practices in place to provide services and resources to family caregivers and people with disabilities.

Since the work of a caregiver is so essential to the well-being of a care recipient, it is quite obvious that keeping a care recipient in the care of a wholly unqualified or abusive caregiver is very dangerous for the care recipient, and in cases of patients with violent tendencies, for the caregiver too.

Caregiver abuse refers to physical or mental maltreatment of a vulnerable care recipient by a caregiver, which often results in mental, emotional, sexual, or physical injury. Abuse of a care recipient by a caregiver can take on many forms. A caregiver may refuse to feed a care recipient or may deprive the recipient of needed medication, thereby keeping the recipient in perpetual pain or discomfort. Abuse can also take physical form by way of hitting or infliction of bodily injury, and it can include verbal assault or even isolation (locking up a care recipient in a room for several consecutive hours, for instance). Caregiver abuse can occur anywhere, at home, in the clinic, at adult daycare centers, or even at retirement homes for the elderly. Abuse of care recipients can also be inflicted by anybody, from highly trusted family members to paid professional caregivers. According to the state statute on caregiver abuse, "abuse" means the intentional infliction of bodily injury on an incapacitated adult. "Bodily injury," on the other hand, means substantial physical pain, illness, or any impairment of physical condition. "Caregiver" refers to any person who has assumed legal responsibility or contractual obligation for the care of an incapacitated adult. The term 'caregiver' also refers to facilities operated by private or public agencies, organizations, or institutions which provide services to, and have assumed responsibility for, the care of an incapacitated adult.

"Incapacitated adult" means any person eighteen years of age or older who by reason of advanced age or physical, mental, or other infirmity is unable to carry on the daily activities of life necessary to sustain life and reasonable health.

According to the above definitions, a caregiver who abuses an incapacitated adult or who knowingly permits another person to abuse an incapacitated adult is guilty of a misdemeanor, and upon conviction thereof, shall be fined or confined in jail for not less than ninety days or more than one year, or both fined and confined, depending on the actual offense committed.

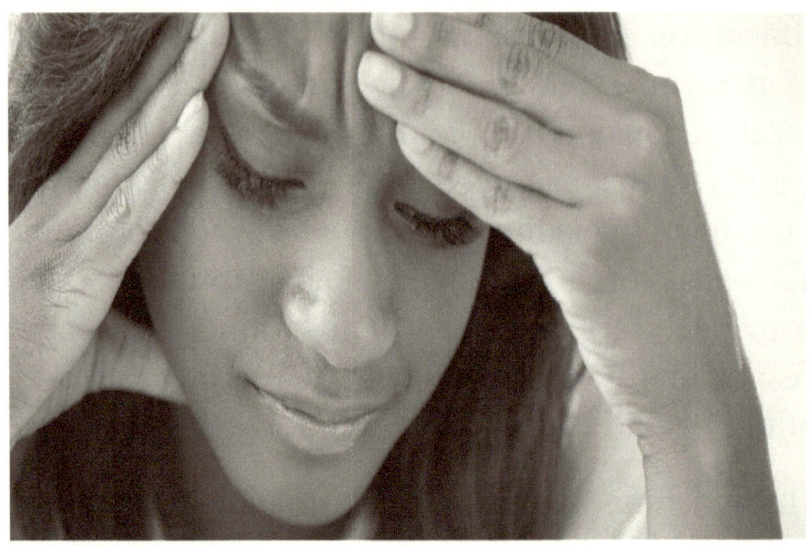

One of the most common factors responsible for caregiver or elder abuse today is caregiver stress and related problems, which affect the ability of caregivers to properly care for their patients. Other factors, such as substance abuse or financial frustration, can also lead to caregiver abuse in many different settings. While it must be noted that caregivers have no excuse whatsoever for their maltreatment of innocent care recipients, it should also be considered that taking care of a disabled person can be a very stressful and challenging process and can evoke different responses from different people in the long run. In a nutshell, not everybody can perfectly fit into the role of an informal caregiver, especially if the care recipient is not a blood relative and if the financial compensation involved does not match the value of the services being rendered.

To help reduce the incidence of caregiver abuse among informal and professional caregivers, issues relating to intense physical and emotional stress should be addressed at all times, which is one of the primary reasons I have written this book. When a caregiver is less stressed, he/she will be in a better position to care for a patient. Apart from excessive stress, as stated earlier, financial constraints can cause issues like anxiety, depression, and other psychological problems. Aggrieved caregivers may take their anger or anxiety out on care recipients, leading to ugly incidents of caregiver abuse.

Caregiver abuse usually begins with steadily increasing anxiety and stress levels, as caregivers begin to feel helpless and trapped in their unwanted situations. With time, these caregivers may begin to see their care recipients as a burden, causing resentment when they require assistance. If caregiver abuse goes unchecked, the care recipient may end up terribly injured or emotionally devastated before other people realize what's going on. If the abusive caregiver is a sibling caregiver who lives alone with his challenged care recipient, caregiver abuse can take an extreme, deadly form, and friends and neighbors may not realize what's going on in time to save the care recipient. In cases where the recipient is non-verbal, he or she may have to suffer caregiver abuse from a family caregiver for years before getting the needed help. If a family caregiver engages in substance abuse or consumes alcohol in excessive quantities, the chances of caregiver abuse occurring increase.

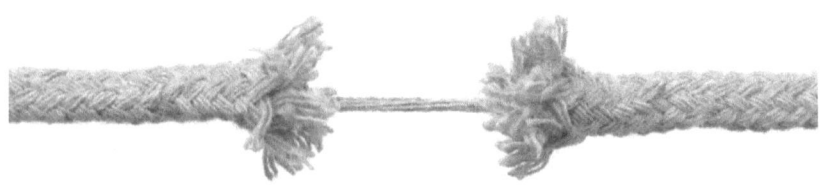

To help prevent caregiver abuse, it is important for caregivers to manage their stress levels. Online and physical community support groups can go a long way in helping to reduce stress levels by providing resources, advice, and assistance to strung out caregivers. Stress-reducing activities like yoga and exercise can also help managing the hardships of caregiving. In extreme cases of caregiver stress, counseling and rehabilitation for caregivers who are addicted to drugs may be a necessary course of action to help prevent or curb caregiver abuse.

If family and friends find out that a sibling caregiver is abusing his or her care recipient, they can come together to help manage the caregiver's burdens. If the situation does not improve, then the care recipient should be removed from the caregiver's custody.

If you are a sibling or informal caregiver, you may want to take a look at these following questions and answer them to the best of your ability:

Caregiver Kudos:

- A. What are some of your strengths as a caregiver?

- B. What are some of your weaknesses as a caregiver?

- C. Even without formal training, what is the one caregiver duty you can perform with ease?

CHAPTER 6: RESOURCES

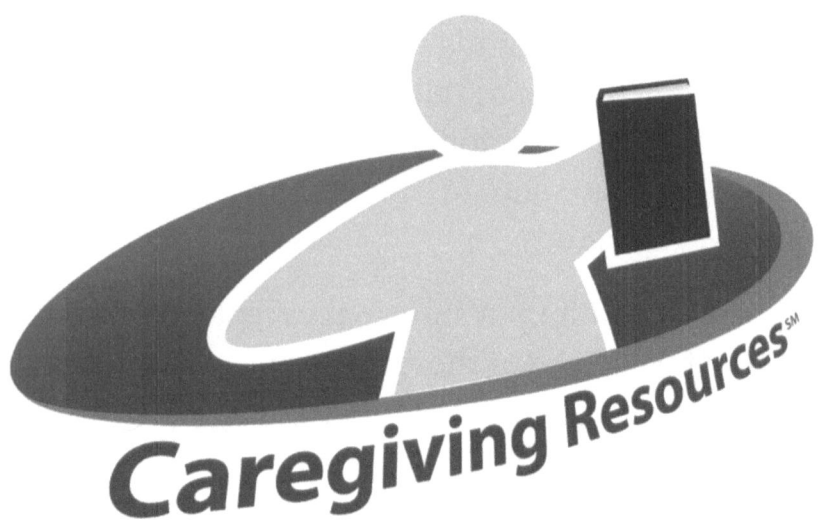

A resource is something used to achieve an objective. When caring for care recipients, informal caregivers need all the help they can get to effectively manage the health of their charges and see to the recipient's general well-being. Apart from helping to improve the quality of life of care recipients, facilities have also been put in place by the State and several non-profit organizations to help improve the standard of living of informal and paid caregivers, with resources made available to make their job easier.

Sibling Caregiver

The first and perhaps most important resource any sibling caregiver can have at his disposal is a host of well-meaning friends and loyal, helpful family members. The work of a caregiver is quite stressful, from having to move the care recipient around the house all day, to fixing his meals and feeding him, administering medication, entertaining the care recipient, listening to the recipient voice his fears if he is verbal... the list is endless. The work of a caregiver takes an intense physical and emotional toll on the caregiver, and if the caregiver does not get the appropriate rest, he or she may succumb to the pressure and break down. If the caregiver feels too stressed or feels overly pressured, he/she may resort to substance abuse, which will in turn affect the care recipient. And if intervention is not sought right away, the care recipient may sustain serious injuries, or, in extreme cases, lose his/her life.

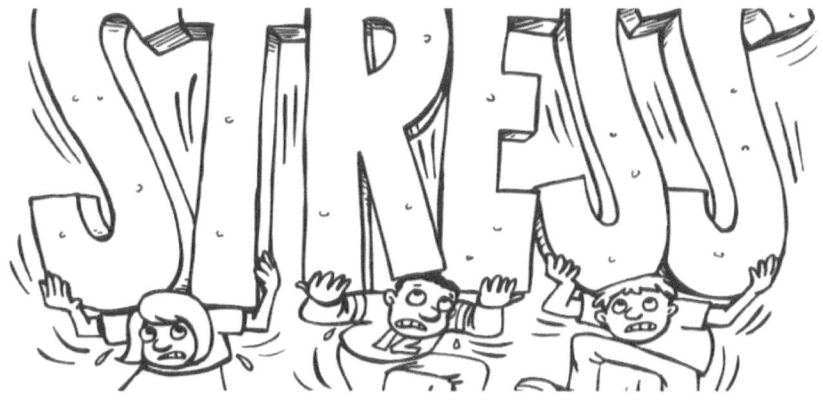

Therefore, it is imperative that caregivers seek the help of a trusted family member or friend before stress gets out of hand. If possible, researchers recommend that the caregiver and care recipient take a vacation at least once or twice a year. This would help both the caregiver and care recipient to unwind, learn new things, and create new experiences in a different environment. Periodic vacations may help improve the mental health of patients with specific disorders. Caregivers, especially informal and unpaid caregivers, are advised to fit some well needed rest into their routines as often as possible. A stressed caregiver is a huge liability to himself, his care recipient, and society at large.

Information is power. When caregivers are appropriately informed about the opportunities available to help make their work easier, it can go a long way in helping to improve the quality of the services they render. As mentioned earlier, technology has helped to change the world in so many ways, many of which couldn't even be imagined years ago. Today, caregivers with access to internet-enabled devices can easily search for available resources to help them do their work better and make life easier for their care recipients. If the available information about a particular resource is not exhaustive enough to be worked with, caregivers can find time when they are not taking care of their care recipients to inquire about available resources at specified social service offices.

A county social service office sees to the management of social services in a particular community or region. Social services are a range of public services provided by the government and by private and non-profit organizations. These public services aim to create more effective organizations, build stronger communities, and promote equality and opportunity. Social services include benefits and facilities such as education, food subsidies, healthcare, police, fire services, and so on. For a caregiver seeking help, the local social services office is a great place to start. Inquiries can be made about options available to make caregiving easier and less taxing, and information about other organizations that handle issues related to social resources can be obtained.

To ease the strain on caregivers and help improve the quality of care received by care recipients, a growing number of private and public organizations are springing up, offering home- and community-based caregiving services. Most of these services are geared towards solving long-term care issues. The goal is usually to relieve the caregiver of some of his/her routine duties.

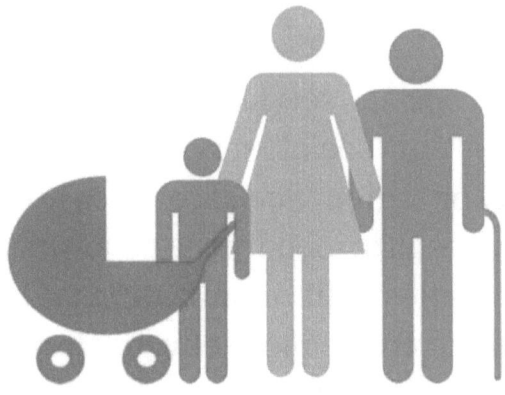

Information about these organizations can be found from local social service offices, and caregivers all over the world are taking advantage of the quality services provided by these organizations to reduce stress and learn useful caregiving practices. Most of the services rendered by these organizations are provided by nurses, trained aids, and trusted volunteers who have been certified as professionals in their field; therefore, caregivers and families of care recipients have nothing to worry about when it comes to the quality of the service they receive. The provided services usually range from household chores to in-house medical care, and these organizations may come to help out up to two times a week, depending on the care recipient's needs, location, and a few other factors. Some professional organizations also offer periodic caregiver help services and in-house medical examinations for disabled patients for a subscription fee. Depending on the condition of the care recipient and how in-need the family is, these paid professional organizations can offer all sorts of services at the residence of the care recipient. They can also assist in taking the care recipient on a vacation, a trip, or out and about in the community. Their main aim is to take care of disabled, elderly, and other special needs people for a fee.

COMPANIONSHIP SERVICES

Companionship services are usually rendered by local agencies that provide affordable service whereby care recipients are matched with experienced psychological experts who have volunteered to help encourage and keep care recipients company periodically. These companions also help with home supervision, reassurance, and friendly social interactions. Frequent visits from a dedicated companion can help ease the stress on a caregiver and can help to enhance the mental health and psychological well-being of a care recipient.

HOUSEKEEPING SERVICES

General housekeeping and upkeep services are usually rendered by a special group of volunteers in some states. Most of the volunteers are not trained medical or psychological experts, but they get together regularly to help ease the burden on caregivers by taking on tasks such as laundry, cooking, errands, and shopping. Some of these volunteers include homemakers and home care aides. These volunteers also provide help with the bathing and dressing of the care recipient. For general home upkeep, there are home repair services that perform minor maintenance and repairs. These volunteers usually offer their services free of charge, but some organizations also render these services for a fee. Your local social services center may be able to point you in the direction of some of these services.

MEAL PREP SERVICES

Occasionally, my brother works with volunteers to take food to the elderly. Preparing meals on a daily basis can become very stressful for caregivers, and care recipients may not be able to provide much assistance with fixing the meals. Therefore, there may come a time when meal delivery services will be needed by the caregiver or the care recipient. In some states, volunteers get together during their free time to cook and distribute food packs to care recipients and senior citizens and their caregivers. These volunteers also visit retirement homes and residential facilities for the physically challenged to help play their part in the development of society. The services provided by these volunteers is also usually free of charge, but professional organizations that deliver meals based on a daily schedule also exist to help ease the burden on family caregivers.

RESPITE SERVICES/ COMMUNITY LIVING

In situations where caregivers, for one reason or another, have to leave their care recipient for an extended period of time, residential homes for the physically challenged exist to help caregivers take care of their challenged loved ones while they are away. These residential homes usually have standby medical services available, and dedicated professional caregivers and nurses are usually available around the clock to tend to the residents. Wholesome meals and comfortable accommodation are usually offered to the enrolled care recipients, and constant attention is always paid to each recipient to help mold them into useful members of their society, despite their disability. These residential homes also organize fun activities like trips, games, and sporting events to help make the residents feel as normal as possible and to help enhance their psychomotor skills. Some residential facilities offer special classes for children and adults with learning disabilities to acquire basic educational knowledge and vocational skills to help them integrate well into society when the time comes. Periodic health screenings are often available at these facilities, too.

TRANSPORTATION SERVICES

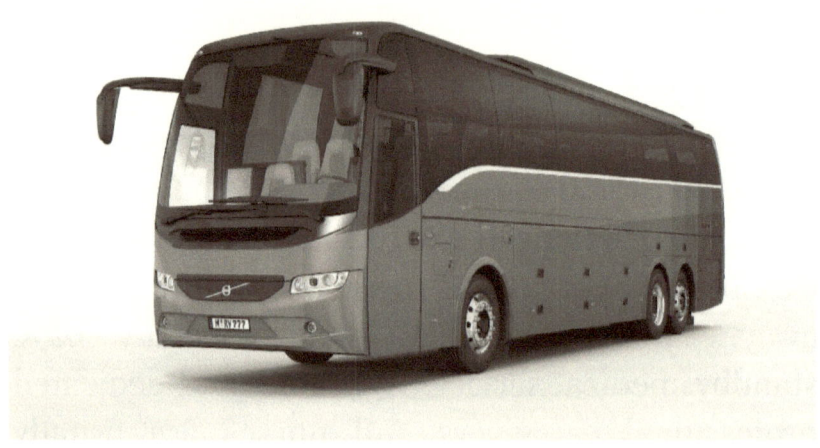

As a caregiver, if you and your loved one need to get to a particular location, i.e., for a trip, a medical consultation, or for your day-to-day activities, dedicated transport services provided by the State, county, or borough are available to you. To seek the services of these transportation agencies, reaching out to your case manager or local social services office is your best bet. These Access Rides or services vehicles are wheelchair accessible, relieving the caregiver of the physical stress associated with moving a care recipient around. They can also help alleviate the emotional stress that arises from the stigmatization of challenged citizens by the general public. Some of these transport agencies also offer assistance with transfers, use of hoists and mobility aids, personal care needs, periodic assistance with transport to medical care appointments, and full career support at sporting events.

Several transport agencies for the disabled offer their services at affordable rates, and if needed, periodic subscriptions can be paid often by the State through Medicaid. When you enroll your loved one to be part of these transportation services, it could take a while for you to get comfortable allowing them to ride alone with the driver or with other care recipients. If this is the case, feel free to accompany your sibling or care recipient to wherever he/she needs to be, so that you may gauge the quality of the service provided by the transport agency and ensure the safety and comfort of your loved one.

HOW TO BOOK A RIDE

Booking the services of these transport agencies has become easier over the years. Most times, all you have to do is register online by providing your personal information and that of your care recipient, the nature of the disability, and your residential address. Once this is done, you can order a ride when needed, or pay a subscription for periodic pickups. Be sure to contact your case manager to find out how Medicad can cover the cost. For some transport agencies, mobile applications are available to improve the ease of hailing a ride for a disabled care recipient. Apart from affordability and privacy, another good reason to patronize a dedicated transport agency for physically challenged citizens is that their vehicles are usually specifically retro-fitted for citizens in wheelchairs, and emergency medical services may be provided on board. Therefore, convenience and functionality are other cogent reasons to use a dedicated transport agency.

ADULT DAY CARE CENTERS

Obligations an informal caregiver has will require leaving their care recipient for hours at a time. Be it school, work, stress, or simply needing a break, caregivers do need time to themselves, which is why adult day cares are a life saver!

An adult day care is used to relieve the caregiver of his or her duties for the day while ensuring that the care recipient will still receive the proper care in a safe, friendly environment. These centers usually operate during normal business hours five days a week.

Adult day care centers provide quality meals, meaningful educational and vocational activities, and general supervision. The care provided is often focused on socialization and provision of quality medical care in order to improve participants' health and guide their progress in the right direction. Most adult day care centers focus on providing care for people with specific chronic conditions such as Alzheimer's disease and other related forms of dementia. Their services may also be available for any adult with disabilities and also the elderly population. Numerous centers maintain a nurse on-site and devote a room for participants who require their vital signs to be checked and evaluated regularly. External medical personnel are also usually provided regularly to attend to special medical needs of patients. Some adult day care centers may also provide facilities for transportation and personal care, including support groups for caregivers. In the field of transportation aid for care recipients, some well-established adult day care centers have a transport services section that picks up regular patrons from their homes every day at a scheduled time and returns these patrons back to their homes at the end of the day. Their caregivers must be present in the evenings to receive their loved one. It is usually more convenient to use the transport service provided by these care centers, as their vehicles have been modified to cater to the needs of the disabled, and the safety and comfort of care recipients are assured.

Attending adult day care centers can prevent care recipients from needing constant external medical attention, as the activities and routine medical care received at these centers can go a long way in helping to enhance the well-being of the care recipient and also help in the quick detection and treatment of any ailments or diseases. For visitors who would otherwise stay at home alone, social stimulation and recreational activities have been known to help improve or maintain physical and cognitive functions. The more severe the disease, the greater the burden is on the caregiver, and the more relieving it becomes to have the care recipient attend an adult day care center.

All certified adult day care centers are monitored and staffed for the protection of participants. These facilities also help attend to the needs of new care recipients who are having trouble connecting with others, or patrons who do not feel comfortable in certain environments. Such programs aim to build up confidence and the ability to maintain an independent lifestyle along with improving physical and mental health.

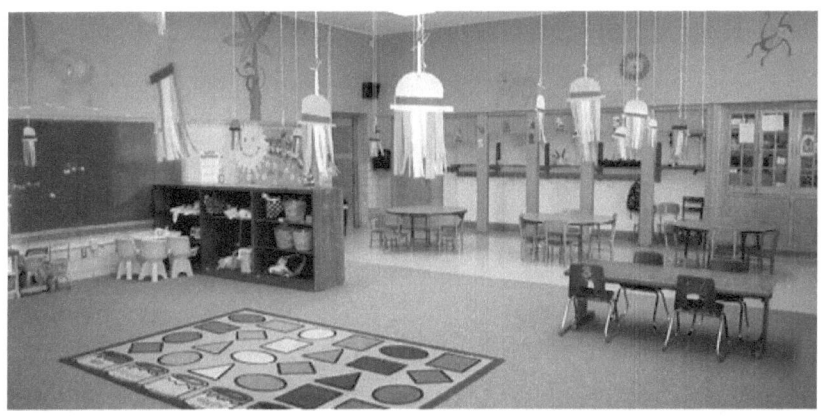

Another important aspect of professional adult day care centers is the fact that challenged patrons have access to medically-recommended diets, which can help to mitigate the effects of their disorders and help them improve their overall health. These day care centers can also provide caregivers with information about healthy diet plans and exercise regimens, which can be followed to help patients with particular disorders. For participants who are just coming from rehabilitation or dementia wards, adult day care center routines may help make sure that needed medication is taken at appropriate times, as the patrons are under supervision. They can also help patients improve their mental health through regular visits by a qualified psychological expert. Healthy, fun activities are usually an integral part of the schedules of most adult day care centers, helping participants discover themselves, relate better with other members of society, build self-confidence, boost their self-esteem, and pick new interests or hobbies, which can go a long way in improving their overall health.

Adult day care centers have expanded over the last few decades, because the healthcare services currently available in them far surpass those of any other time. As these centers become more in-demand, more regions in the United States are experiencing a rapid increase in the numbers of them available. The main and common aim of all adult day care centers around the world is to provide quality care to and enriching interactions with other participants. Adult day care centers help participants to develop a positive outlook on life and maximize the opportunities they have to make positive impacts on their societies. The skill and knowledge levels of autistic people who attend adult day care centers have been proven to far exceed those of adults on the spectrum who don't. Activities commonly engaged in by participants include arts and crafts, music, games like bingo and scrabble, exercise activities like yoga, interesting discussion, general socialization, and conversations intended to form friendly relationships.

Adult day care centers also help to promote independence and free thinking for people with physical and learning disabilities and aged citizens. The purpose of this is to introduce them back into normal social environments and to help them gain new friends and skillsets. Today in the United States, there are over 5000 registered adult day service centers providing care for over 300,000 elderly and disabled citizens each day. About half of the adult day care centers available in the United States exist as profit-oriented organizations. Daily fees may be less than a home health visit, and half the cost of a skilled nursing facility, but fees vary depending on the services provided. The average daily cost of adult day care services in the United States is $70, with funding mostly coming from participant fees, third-party insurance, and public and philanthropic sources.

With more people needing assistance and guidance to enter the world again after injuries, illnesses, or long-term chronic disorders, there is additional demand for adult day care facilities. With the variety of programs such centers have in place, participants have a much better chance of achieving their goals and living better, more fulfilled lives. Statistically, about 19.1% of caregivers opt for adult day care centers to help relieve themselves of the repeated stress of caring for their challenged loved one.

Faith communities and religious organizations are another important resource available to caregivers all over the world. Many caregivers everywhere are seeking and finding help from established religious networks, who usually help caregivers with financial assistance and aid in the form of food and medical assistance. These religious communities may actually own well-established healthcare facilities that are open to the general public, but with special sections dedicated to the care of physically challenged patients and people with chronic disorders. When the appropriate appeals are placed to religious leaders, healthcare facilities owned by faith communities may be accessed for free, and quality medication may also be administered free of charge, provided that the religious institution is satisfied that the caregiver or recipient does not intend to use the medication for any other purpose than treating the challenged person.

Religious institutions also help to alleviate the stress experienced by caregivers in the discharge of their caregiving duties. At regular intervals, meetings at religious centers may be organized by the centers themselves to help educate attendees on how to better care for their care recipients and better utilize available technology for that purpose. Special donations received from well-meaning members of the religious community may also be channeled into the care of challenged members of these same communities. Donations may be used for the purchase of wheelchairs for immobilized members, for instance, or a special fund may be set up for the establishment of a dedicated adult day care center with experienced medical personnel to account for the daily needs of disabled members of religious communities.

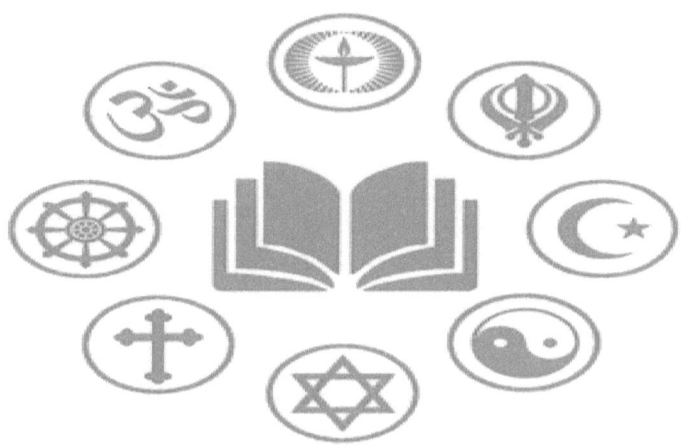

THE CARE ACT - CAREGIVER, ADVISE, RECORD, ENABLE

One of the most pressing difficulties that informal caregivers all over the world must regularly cope with is the issue of financial constraints. According to research, a considerable percentage of care recipients with physical disabilities and cognitive disorders live below the poverty line. This discovery means that more energy and attention needs to be paid to the financial well-being of caregivers and care recipients all over the world. To help ease constraints on the families of physically disabled patients, most states in the United States have adopted a policy to pay informal caregivers for work provided.

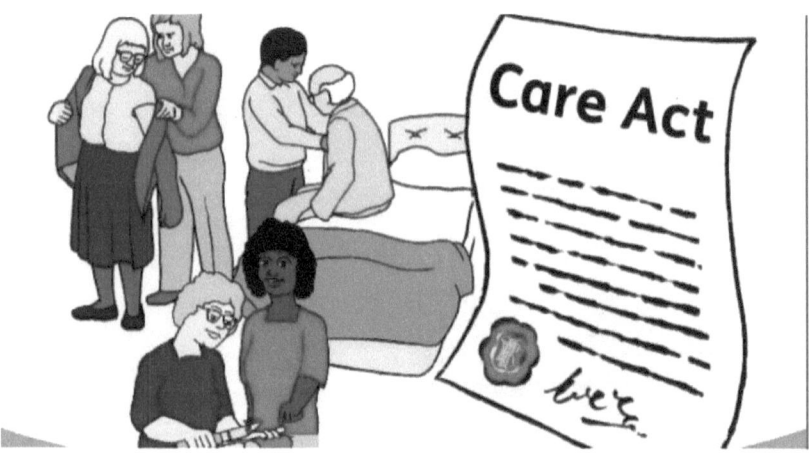

In the United States, the CARE Act supports family caregivers when a loved one goes into the hospital, and it helps the caregiver to learn what must be done to safely provide care when their loved one is discharged home.

The CARE Act informational wallet card can be downloaded for free on the AAR website and printed for caregivers and their loved ones for reference purposes. The CARE Act improves coordination and communication between family caregivers, their loved ones/patients, and hospitals. It does this through three main provisions.

Designation: The hospital must make provisions for the patient to record the name of a family caregiver into his/her medical record upon admission to the hospital.

Notification: The hospital must inform the family caregiver if the loved one is to be transferred to another healthcare facility or back home if the patient is not competent to be moved.

Explanation: The hospital must explain in detail all the medical tasks – such as medication management, injections, and injury care – that the family caregiver would have to perform at home when the hospital deems it necessary.

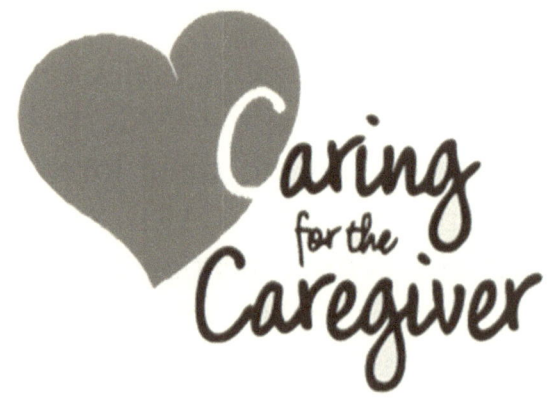

Caring for the Caregiver

Caregivers need to understand that while laws and policies have been implemented to help improve the general quality of healthcare delivery and the financial well-being of caregivers and challenged persons all over the world, some bureaucratic setbacks can occur in the course of a caregiver trying to take advantage of a purely legal opportunity.

As mentioned earlier, when the financial obligation of serving as a caregiver becomes too uncomfortable, help can be sought from appropriate sources: from friends and family, from designated public and private institutions, from dedicated programs created by corporate bodies, and from research institutes who can help with medication and healthcare needs. Being a caregiver is quite difficult, and you deserve to get all the help you need.

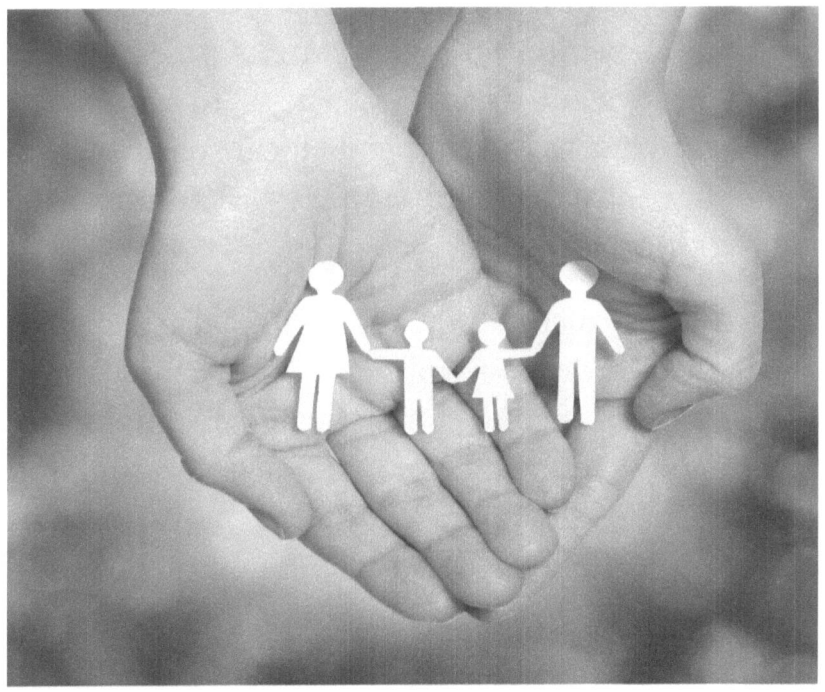

In the United States, there is a support mechanism for caregivers who care for people above the age of 60 years. The Older Americans Act Amendments of 2000 established and funded the National Family Caregiver Support Program (NFCSP). The program was created to help relieve the financial hardships involved with continual care by family caregivers (of any age) who act as unpaid caregivers for loved ones 60 or older. It is also possible for informal caregivers to get paid for their work, depending on the state. I did get paid for caring for my brother, because it was a full-time job. I didn't know such a possibility existed until his social worker mentioned it to me. These types of resources are available depending on your state. As a caregiver, you can begin your journey to financial empowerment by visiting your local social service center or a local disability center to ask for more in-depth information.

The use of technology, as stated earlier, has changed the way the world works in many ways. With the aid of new, sophisticated technological equipment, caregivers can lessen the accumulated stress caused by their job of looking after and caring for a challenged loved one. Equipment such as webcams or closed-circuit television can be used for remote monitoring of sibling care recipients. This can enable real-time monitoring from a close-by or remote location. The use of these cameras can also enable multi-tasking. The caregiver can keep an eye on the care recipient while doing something else within the house. Revolutions in the field of Artificial Intelligence have also helped to reduce stress and exhaustion experienced by caregivers in the discharge of their duties. For example, Amazon's new artificial intelligence robot, Alexa, which is incorporated into Amazon Echo, can control smart devices through voice commands and can perform tasks related to home automation.

It can even order pizza! Therefore, with this kind of technology in place, mobile care recipients can manage alone for a few hours, although constant help may still be required in some circumstances. When care recipients need help, they can simply place a call entirely with their voices, without touching their phones.

When caregivers are paid well and have access to stress-alleviating equipment and resources, they can focus on attending to the needs of those under their care. When a comfortable and less-frustrating environment is provided for a caregiver to work in, stress levels are likely to drop, along with the chances of caregiver abuse.

Another benefit of technology to caregivers is access to support groups, which have been instrumental to many types of support workers over the years. With the help of a group of caregivers who have a wealth of experience, a new caregiver can receive insight on how to navigate the world of caregiving. Support groups can help a caregiver more easily access available aids and financial help, which may be quite difficult otherwise. Having friends that understand your journey and the ups and downs of caregiving is why these types of support groups make a difference. Sometimes, a problem discussed with the right person means a problem half-solved. So, it is advisable for all caregivers to join some sort of support group, be it online or at a physical location, as it will make a world of difference.

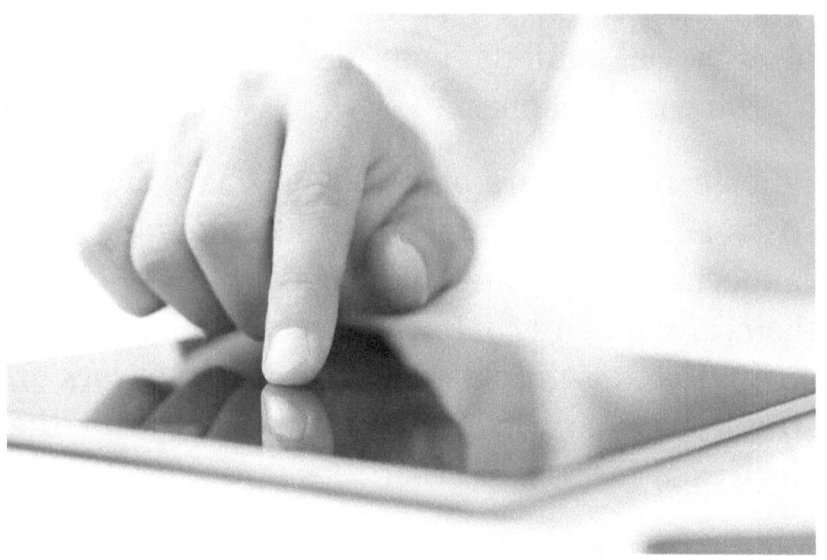

THE IMPACT ETHNICITY, RELIGION, AND SEXUAL ORIENTATION HAVE ON CAREGIVING

In most cultures and religions all over the world, taking care of a challenged family member is perceived as a good deed or an honorable act. In most of these cultures, getting paid for taking care of a disabled family member is viewed as absurd, and caregivers are expected to give everything to their care recipients without complaining. However, most of these cultures and religions do not take into consideration the intense stress and exhaustion that comes with being an informal caregiver. Therefore, most local family caregivers who belong to minority ethnic groups or who live in strongly culturally-inclined communities have to bear the challenges and complications associated with being a caregiver in silence, without earning a dime even when they are entitled to it.

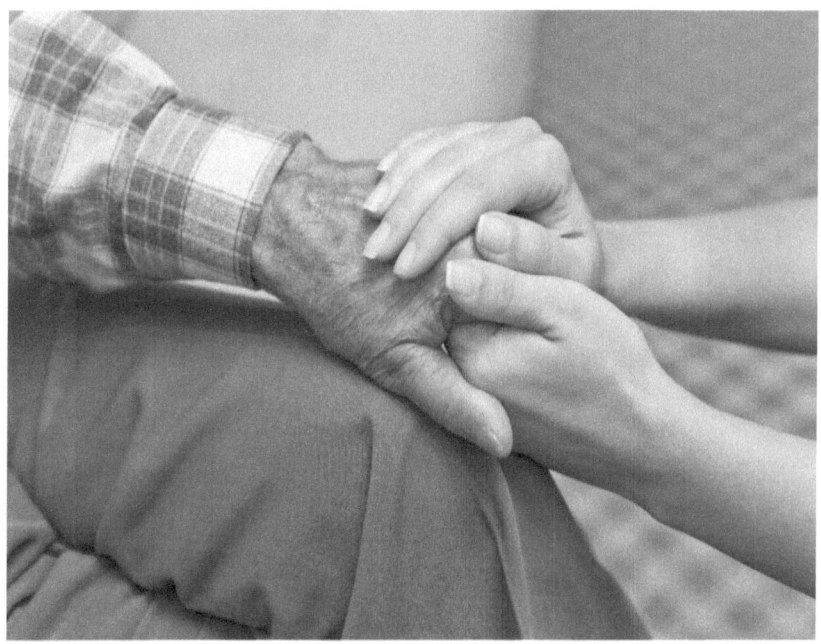

Caregivers, care recipients, and the public should be properly educated and informed about the work that caregivers do, the scope of their responsibilities, and the intense tolls that their responsibilities can have on their health. Caregivers really deserve to be paid, and they shouldn't be denied this right simply because of cultural or religious beliefs. As a matter of fact, the general public should be sensitized to compensating caregivers in cash, and in kind, with moral support, and in any other way possible, to help encourage them to take better care of their care recipients and to help build a healthier, happier society.

Discrimination and stigmatization of certain categories of people is a menace that needs to come to an end. Some of the most stigmatized and alienated people in the world today are care recipients suffering from physical and cognitive disabilities. The world needs to treat disabled people better. As a fully healthy individual, you do not need to see a disabled person as a lesser individual solely because you can speak, and he is non-verbal. Society needs to advocate for the equality of disabled and able-bodied individuals. Apart from regular care recipients and their caregivers, another group of people seriously discriminated against all over the world are members of the LGBT (Lesbian, Gay, Bisexual, and Transgender) community. People with unconventional sexual orientations should be accommodated more often within society. Gay people should not be denied opportunities, kicked out of place, or denied help because of their sexual orientation. We have advanced to a level where everybody should have equal opportunities and chances, and sexual orientation should be the last thing used to judge a person's character. Members of the LGBT community need to be accepted into society as anyone else, and gay caregivers and their care recipients should be afforded all the opportunities available to regular caregivers and their challenged loved ones.

On several occasions, caregivers of those in the LGBT (lesbian, gay, bisexual and transgender) community have reported being denied help and financial assistance by administrators who have found little ways of disqualifying them. Legislation alone cannot solve these problems. Online and offline training seminars and talks that appeal to a listener's sense of reason should be targeted at 'anti-gay' people. Also, avenues should be made available for challenged gay patients to report any maltreatment experienced at the hands of public service workers as a direct result of their sexual orientation.

Challenged gay people and their caregivers should also have access to the proper channels for sourcing information and financial aid. They should be encouraged to speak up against discrimination and demand their rights, even in the face of stigmatization. If we are going to build a world that is just, fair, and truly free, we all need to understand that everybody, able-bodied or disabled, gay or straight, needs to be given equal chances to pursue their dreams.

A good caregiver is a well-informed caregiver. Caregivers should endeavor to be well informed at all times so that they may take better care of their challenged care recipients and make their own jobs as caregivers easier and less stressful.

Now that we've talked about a few resources and the consequences of their lack, here are a few questions for you to ponder and take action on.

A. How accessible are resources in your community? List a few of the resources you use and tweet us @thenewswithOB using the hash tag #whoisaSiblingcaregiver

B. If you got the runaround, did you give up? What did you do to make sure that you and your loved one got the service you needed?

Do you have a fallback plan in case the resources you depend on are no longer available? If not, what plans are you working on to ensure there is a plan B in place?

CHAPTER 7:
ADVICE TO PARENTS

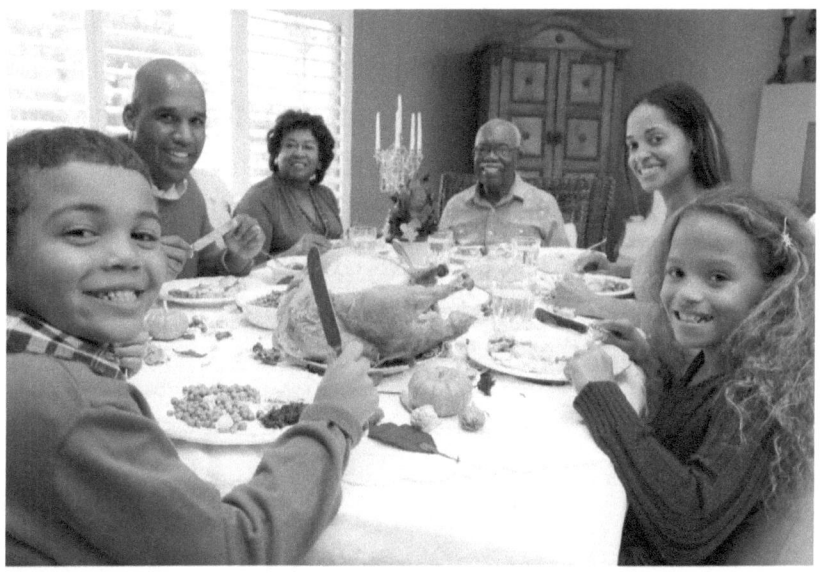

Finding out that your loved one or friend has developed a chronic condition or cognitive disorder can be quite painful. However, finding out that your own kid is autistic can also be very traumatizing. In the first few months after making this discovery, you may actually need professional help to get you through the challenge of finding out your little one will likely require lifelong special attention. This is where most parents first get it wrong. As soon as their suspicions regarding their child being autistic are confirmed, people have been known to break down in tears and sink deeper into the throes of depression with every passing day as the reality of the permanence of their child's condition begins to sink in. To prevent these kinds of occurrences, it is important for parents of autistic children (especially if the child is their first) to seek professional help for themselves, so that they can remain emotionally stable. Qualified therapists will come in very handy helping young parents to get through the painful realization that their child has cognitive deficiencies.

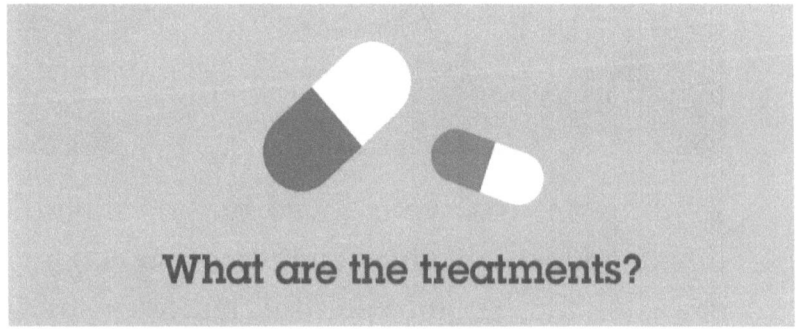

What are the treatments?

After discovering that your child has a learning/developmental disability, the most important thing is to discuss the available treatment options with a seasoned expert in the field of pediatric medicine. Your healthcare expert can help you choose a treatment plan or suggest useful medical procedures to help your child if the disability was diagnosed soon enough. As awkward as this seems, a lot of parents, overcome by the grief and pain of realizing that their child is autistic, actually fail to pursue the possibility of mitigating the condition by finding quality medical care. As a parent seeking help for an autistic child, your personal mantra must be to "never give up, never back down." If you hear about a helpful treatment regimen being practiced somewhere, please follow up and check it out.

As a parent, you need to properly understand the nature of your child's disability. It is also very important to note that the fact that your child is autistic does not necessarily mean that your child will turn out a failure. Although approximately 40% of autistic children are non-verbal, this does not mean that autistic children do not understand language; therefore, you have to be extremely careful about the words you utter around your autistic children. Many suicide cases involving autistic children have been recorded all over the world, and research has proven that social rejection and alienation of these kids, even at home, is the primary reason for such suicides among children with cognitive disorders. Parents also need to understand the strengths and weaknesses of their autistic kids. The autism spectrum disorder includes genetic impairments that actually make some autistic children incredibly gifted, with skills that enable them to excel beyond imagination in tasks requiring excellent visual skills and in fields like music, mathematics, and art. In a study conducted among some children with symptoms of autistic spectrum disorder, it has been found that many autistic children actually have outstanding musical capabilities. One autistic boy was so talented in the arts that he had some of his paintings exhibited by the time he was 10.

Research has shown that most normal people cannot commit a string of more than ten to fifteen numbers to memory at a stretch, but some autistic children with special mathematical skills have been known to calculate square roots of up to six-digit numbers in a matter of seconds. These kids can commit a large amount of information to memory at once, and they can execute complex mental processes at unbelievable speeds. Therefore, while your kid may be autistic, he isn't necessarily dull! Mentally gifted autistic kids have been known to bag college degrees at as little as 14 years of age, scoring in the 90th percentile in subjects ranging from the arts and music to advanced mathematics all through their stints at schools for the gifted.

Sibling Caregiver

One of the reasons postulated for the impressive mental abilities in autistic children is their unusual ability to focus and pay extreme attention to detail. While normal kids are likely to have multiple streams of thought running through their minds at once, these gifted autistic children focus on just one line of thought and concentrate intensely, harnessing the power granted to them by their autistic spectrum disorder. One of the pointers to realizing your child's strengths as the parent of an autistic kid is to pay very close attention to him or her, note his or her interests and likes. Most autistic children with unusual mental capabilities are obsessive in their interests. By paying close attention to your autistic kid, you can help them appropriately harness their gifts. The bottom line is, not all autistic kids are incapable of coping with serious academic work. Depending on the specific nature of their disorder on the autism spectrum, they may actually be unbelievably good at something that you just haven't realized yet. Do not give up on your kid; pay close attention to him/her and help harness those special abilities before it's too late. In cases of non-verbal autistic children, discovering their interests and special abilities (if any) may be a little more difficult than in their verbal counterparts. As a parent, however, it is your responsibility to watch your children very closely and help them make the best of their lives (even if they aren't autistic!).

Incorporate close friends and family members into the life of your special needs child. This will not only help the child to appreciate the family bond as early as possible, but it will also help you when there is a need to call on a friend or family member for assistance. However, if your child has behavioral problems, it could be difficult to have other people around. That shouldn't stop you. Learn what ticks your child off and how to manage it.

My Child Without Limits is a great online resource that helps families of young children ages 0-5 with developmental delays or disabilities. It is important to seek out professional help for your child at the onset. Research has shown that it is easier to show a special needs child how to do something as opposed to telling them. Below is an excerpt on what goes on in the mind of your child with a disability or developmental delay:

"Show me how to do something rather than just telling me. And be prepared to show me many times. Lots of patience and practice help me learn. Visual supports help me move through

my day. They relieve me of the stress of having to remember what comes next, make for smooth transition between activities, and help me manage my time and meet expectations. I need to see something to learn it, because spoken words are like steam to me; they evaporate in an instant, before I have a chance to make sense of them. I don't have instant-processing skills. Instructions and information presented to me visually can stay in front of me for as long as I need and will be just the same when I come back to them later. Without this, I live with the constant frustration of knowing that I am missing big blocks of information and expectations, and I am helpless to do anything about it."

Taking care of a child with a disability or special needs is no cakewalk for any parent. But it is important not to let the difficulty of being a parent of a disabled child overwhelm you. I know, it is easier said than done, but the truth is, this is a time when the family needs to stick together, especially for the disabled child. Yes, parenting is hard, and doing so for a disabled child is even harder, but make an effort to take the needed breaks, and find time for other members of your family. Ask friends and family to help you, or pay someone trained in the area of your child's special needs to help out for a few hours.

According to recent reports, parents with children who have a disability report more health problems than most other parents the same age. The stress is emotional, physical, and financial. When a parent is raising a child with a disability alone, they can feel that lack of support. A 2008 study published in the journal Qualitative Health Research, following the experiences of 14 parents of children with autism, found that a common feeling was extreme social isolation and a lack of understanding from others. "Group support can offer parents the knowledge, understanding, and acceptance they seek," notes Mary Banach, a professor of social work at the University of New Hampshire. Parents can find comfort, friendship and support in networks like the Autism Support Network, Autism Speaks, and the Autism Society, whose websites provide access to message boards, information about local chapters and meet-ups, and events. I can't emphasize enough the importance of taking a break to avoid burnout. When parents or any caregiver notices anger, guilt, or emotions flying, it is time to stop and ask for help. There are many people out there within your close friends and family willing to help. Don't hesitate to ask.

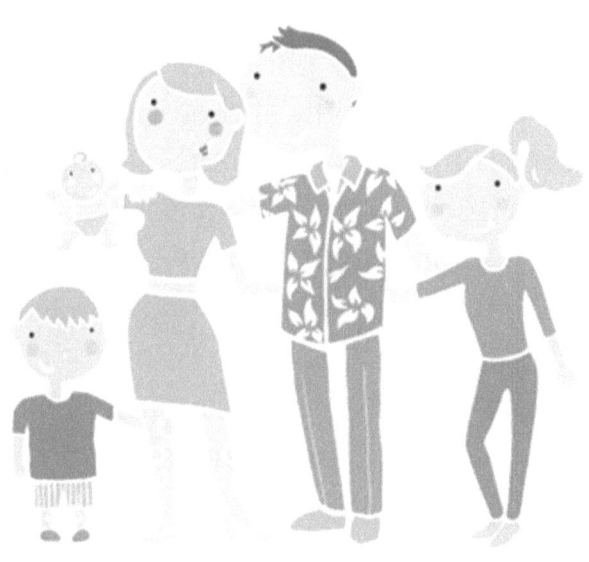

A problem shared is half-solved. So, when you talk about your issues with the right people, helpful solutions and tips emanating from acquired knowledge or experience are likely to be shared, enabling you to handle your situation better and more confidently. Joining a local support group can be a very helpful move for you as a parent. You might wonder, "How can joining a local support group help me take better care of my little one with special needs?"

Well, first of all, from local support groups, you can develop warm companionship and get amazing advice on how to get over the shock that comes with realizing that your child is autistic. Every single member of a local support group is either a parent or guardian to an autistic child like yours, and they perfectly understand what you are going through. Therefore, joining a local support group can give you the companionship you need during your dark days; this is the kind of companionship that you actually need, because it comes from people who truly understand your plight. While it is still important to see a qualified therapist if you think you cannot handle the grief on your own, it also helps a lot to seek consolation from people who have been through exactly your type of situation. So, there is your first reason: emotional support.

Secondly, joining a local support group as the parent of a child who has just been diagnosed with autism can be very helpful for getting tips and more useful information about healthcare practitioners who specialize in dealing with children with autism. Understand that people in these types of support groups are from different backgrounds, and they all have different experiences, so what they have to offer is invaluable. Through trial and error, some of them have managed to find some of the best healthcare facilities available to help care for their autistic children, and their knowledge will help you to do the same. With their help and advice, you will not need any longer to go through the same emotionally-draining stresses of seeking quality healthcare for your own child; they have gone through the stress so that you do not have to.

Closely related to helping you with good healthcare centers, members of local support groups can actually help out with some of the medical procedures that are prescribed by the doctor, usually with your help. At times, as the parent of an autistic child, you just become too emotionally and physically drained to do anything for yourself or your child. To prevent extreme stress, it is important for you to take timely breaks every now and then. Members of local support groups are perfect for this role, because they understand exactly what needs to be done, and they are also well-informed as to what could put your young child in danger. It is still very important, however, to explain any routine procedure that they would be carrying out to them, as described by your healthcare specialist, in case of slight or major differences between what they know and what has been prescribed. Members of your group can also help out periodically with other routine domestic tasks to help ease the burden on you as a family caregiver. While it is very important to talk to your child's pediatrician in the case of any emergency or if you do not understand a particular required procedure, members of your local group can help further explain what the doctor was trying to illustrate by doing it repeatedly in front of you. If the doctor's method of explanation was confusing, or you just weren't in the right frame of mind to absorb the information during the doctor's visit, a member from your support group can certainly help. Remember, they've been down this road before you, or are currently on the same journey with you.

Giving back to society has a way of making us feel fulfilled. Chances are, while you are confronted with the devastating news of your child's diagnosis of autism, society, in the form of local support groups, the local welfare center, the community social service center, and several other support mechanisms, will help you a lot in coping with the news and getting back on your feet. Along the line, you might feel a pressing need to give back to the society that helped you when you were down. In most social support groups, events like charity dinners and yard sales are organized periodically. These events usually bring together the members of these support groups and the other members of their families. These events often serve as a great avenue for other members of the families (including the autistic kids themselves) to interact with other members of the autism community. Fathers, older siblings, and even younger siblings who were probably not part of the support group prior to the event, can come together to share helpful experiences, information, and challenges they have encountered while playing their part in caring for their autistic family members. Best of all, these events can help generate funds, which can be channeled into helping all other autistic children around the world, thereby helping to make the world a better place. Therefore, among other things, your local support group can help a great deal helping you to play your part in giving back to the society that helped you when you needed it most.

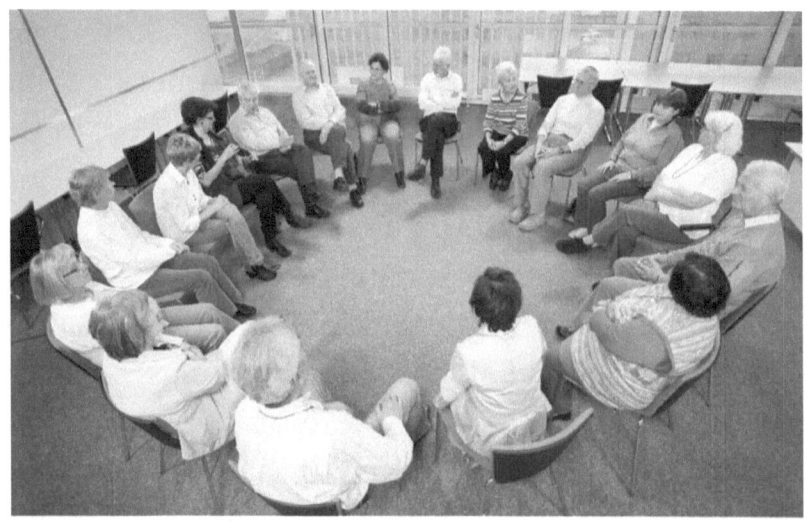

Finally, local support groups can go a long way in helping you get your voice and opinions out into the world. An active local support group can play a huge role in helping you get your grievances and concerns as a parent of an autistic child out to relevant agencies and out to the world as a whole. Targeted campaigns and sensitization programs can be launched to help sensitize other parents, caregivers, and the general public about autism and the great responsibility that rests on the necks of every parent and guardian who is raising an autistic child. These campaigns can also help educate the public about autism and how autistic kids should be accepted as normal members of society. These campaigns can go a long way in helping to curb the stigmatization and alienation of autistic children and their caregivers in society. As a coherent, organized group, a support group for parents raising autistic children can also organize events, such as free medical testing and educational seminars for autistic children and their parents, to help promote the welfare of every stakeholder in the world of autism, and in general to help build a less harsh world for innocent little children.

Online forums are another very important tool that can be used by parents with autistic children to seek useful, quality advice and support, and also to voice their worries. Online forums are usually set up by medical practitioners or experienced caregivers in the autism field to help every struggling parent, sibling, and informal caregiver out there find their way in a world where autism is strongly discriminated against. On these online forums, you can find quality advice and information, you can talk to experts, and you can let out all your pent-up worries to someone who is actually in a position to help you. You can also read about the challenges being faced by parents like you all over the world and what they are doing to solve their problems.

As a parent, it is very important for you to avoid useless and less-driven support groups. Many support groups are established with good intentions, but instead of people coming together to have constructive discussions and organize useful activities, some members just choose to share unimportant information or discuss other issues that cannot in any way help you or your autistic child. These kinds of groups are not really support groups in the true sense of the word; they are just a bunch of people coming together to talk about stuff that tickles their fancies. For your own sake, and to avoid a perpetual waste of time, it would make a lot of sense for you to steer clear of these kinds of gatherings and seek help where you can really get it. If your local support group is not vibrant enough, online forums are always a great alternative for you to get useful information and accurate answers to your burning questions. If there is no support group available at all in your local community, you can set one up yourself and print flyers or posters to generate awareness. You can also set up a personal blog detailing your experience as a parent of a child with Autistic Spectrum Disorder (ASD) to help other people all around the world who are in your shoes find faster and more trustworthy solutions to their parenting challenges.

Sibling Caregiver

As a parent, it is important for you to be as observant as possible for any abnormalities or unusual behaviors in your child. If you notice any signs which are abnormal in your child, it is advisable for you to take them straight to a doctor for examination. Autism is best handled when discovered early. Timely intervention can actually help completely heal autism in some children who do not have it in its chronic form, if the disorder is diagnosed early enough.

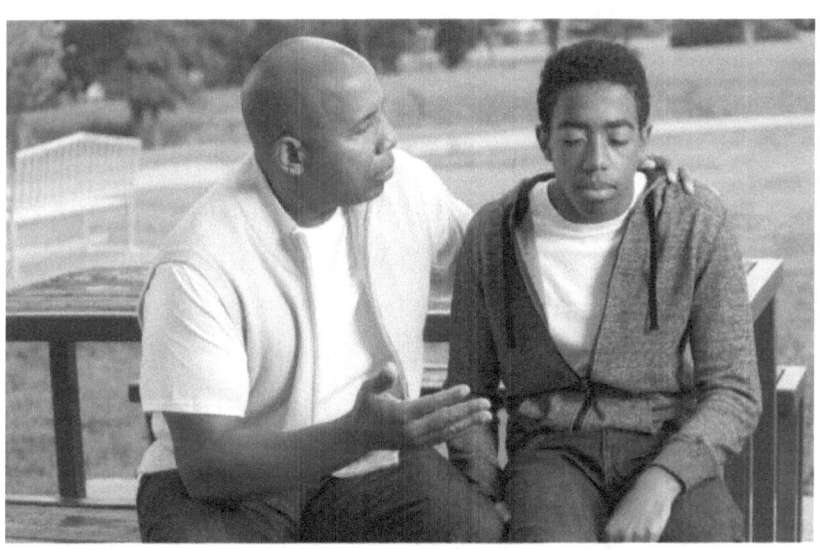

After getting to know about your child's diagnosis, it is important for you to use all practicable means to gain useful knowledge about your child's particular condition. Knowledge empowers, and if you know everything there is to know about your child's condition, you will be in a better position to take proper care of him or her and to discuss your child's treatment options with pediatricians based on the behaviors you have seen him/her exhibit. As the parent of an autistic child, you cannot afford to be laid back, not when their future is at stake. You always have to be on your toes, constantly searching for ways to help your child and understand him or her better. With time, as you continue to research your child's condition, while studying their behavior critically at the same time, you will become an expert on your own child as a particular autistic individual. You would be able to predict some of his actions and reactions to certain variables. As a parent, you must fully understand your child to the very core. Know his quirks, what makes him tick, his interests, likes, and dislikes. Know what makes him throw tantrums, and learn how to gently correct him when he goes wrong. Gaining adequate information about your child and studying his behavioral patterns are both very important duties for you as a good parent to an autistic child.

As a parent, you must learn to be proud of your child at all times, no matter the circumstances. Everybody knows that it is not a walk in the park coming to terms with the fact that your child is autistic. It is decidedly not a piece of cake, either, to introduce your autistic child to your friends from college or high school and say, "Hey, meet my son, Drake. He is autistic." Notwithstanding the social stigma that surrounds your child's condition, as a parent, you must learn to accept your child's condition as an integral part of who he or she is and love him or her unconditionally, regardless of the condition. As a matter of fact, you must especially learn to love them *for* their condition. This is the only way that taunts and alienation issues won't rattle you emotionally. You need to be strong for your child, and to do this, you need to accept and understand his or her condition. Treat him/her gently, watch him/her closely, try to discover his/her interests, and do all you can to help him/her grow and bloom. Since coping with this is not such an easy task, seeing your personal therapist may be a healthy move. However, you must learn to bond and connect with your child on a deep emotional level as soon as possible; see every day as an opportunity for new adventures and discoveries, both for you and for them, and never, ever disparage your child. It ruins their self-worth and self-esteem.

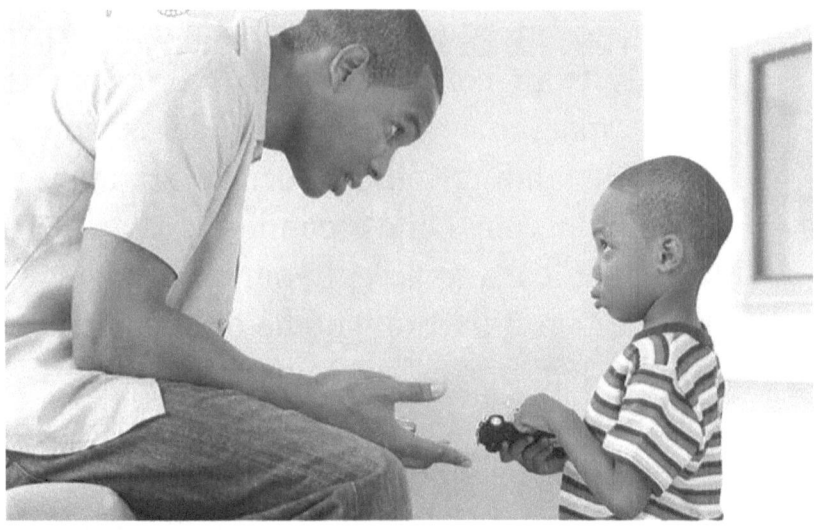

Also, as a parent to an autistic child, one of the important duties you will have to learn is how to imbibe the values of patience and perseverance when dealing with your kid. Most children with cognitive deficiencies find learning this to be an uphill task, especially when it is rushed or presented in a disorganized form. As a parent, you must understand that your child can learn and retain information, just not at the rate which other children do. This is where consistency comes in. While teaching your child to execute a simple task, you must learn to be consistent in your teaching, and try as often as possible to use visual methods of teaching wherever you can. You need to be very patient, calm, and collected, if you hope to help your autistic child learn. Even when they annoy you with their slowness, you must learn to keep a rein on your temper, and slowly repeat and demonstrate the procedure you are trying to teach. Eventually, your little one will learn.

After they have learned simple tasks, it is important to keep things regimented and keep a practicable schedule. Research has proven that autistic children learn and behave better when things follow a regular, predictable pattern. Therefore, as you raise your child, try to set a sort of timetable for the things he does every day, and let a particular order be upheld. If, for instance, he has to brush his teeth first thing in the morning, then take his bath, and then get dressed before eating and heading to school, try to keep this schedule constant. For days like weekends or public holidays, which are exceptions to the normal schedule, you may want to explain to your child in advance why the normal schedule won't be followed those days. Research has also proven that autistic children may find the application of information gained in one environment to a new environment quite challenging. For example, if your child learns a skill in school, and he is not within the school environment, he could find it difficult to apply those skills he had no trouble with before. It is therefore important, in most cases, to explain to your child how to apply what he has learned in one environment in another environment, where the variables are a little different. This would go a long way in helping to enhance your child's mental capabilities.

As an autistic parent, you must learn the importance of helping your child understand the meaning of his actions and the consequences that may result from them. This is where the concept of rewarding your child for good behavior comes in. When trying to inculcate proper social skills in your child, it is important for them to always understand at all times what the gravity of their utterances, actions, inactions, and reactions is. Therefore, when you reward your child for good behavior, it sticks that this particular act earns him a reward, and he should do it more often. When your little one behaves inappropriately, too, it is important to gently reprimand them and have them understand that what they did is not good, or that they could hurt themselves or others while at it. This simple system of rewarding and gently scolding your autistic child can help inculcate model social skills and good behavioral patterns within them. It is necessary, however, to be consistent in your use of the reward and reprimand system. No matter how stressed out or tired you are, if your child has done something deserving a reward, make sure to commend him and let him know he has made you happy. If, on the other hand, he commits an offence, it is important to scold him gently, let him realize why what he did is wrong, let him learn to apologize, and then draw him into your arms and let him know you love him. This helps not only to make your child well-behaved and intelligent, it also helps strengthen the bond you share with him. Above all, spend quality time with your autistic child. Let him understand that he is a big part of your life; let him feel wanted and loved. If he is verbal, let him tell you silly stories, and laugh. Take him on walks to the park or for visits to the zoo. Carefully explain anything he is inquisitive about to him. Having fun will go a long way in helping boost his confidence in you, and will, above all, help him see you as a source of comfort and happiness. What else is the goal of parenting, after all?

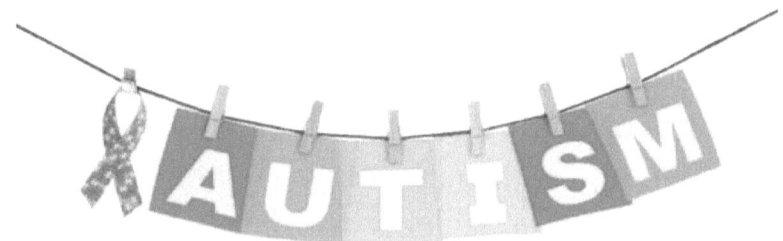

As mentioned earlier, most children with autistic spectrum disorder tend to learn better with the help of visual aids. To help promote the safety of your child within the home, it may be necessary for you to make some demarcations that they can understand and explain the meaning of these demarcations to them. If you only tell them not to touch or carry something without installing any sort of visual reminder for them associated with that object, they can easily forget, and in the end, they might end up injuring themselves or destroying valuable property. It is therefore important for you to install clear, suitable demarcations that can be easily understood. These demarcations will be more effective if your child is present during their installation or even participates in the installation. That way, any time he or she moves close to an object, he/she knows not to touch it because of the presence of the demarcation. It could also be important to explain (with the aid of visual aids, of course) why it might be injurious for your kid to toy with the item in question. That way, you can rest assured that your information has been passed on and retained, and your child's safety is better secured. Suitable demarcations that can be used include bright colorful tapes and warning stickers. However, you should try to watch your child's movements as closely as possible to avoid serious injuries, demarcations or not.

If your autistic little one is non-verbal, communicating and passing information between you might be more difficult. To overcome this, you might need to develop a special kind of sign language to communicate with your child. Doing this can be a thrilling adventure for both of you, as it can be like having a sort of secret code or silent communication. Blinking, looking at your child in a specific way, shaking your head, dancing, screwing up your face, and other kinds of facial and bodily gestures can be very helpful when trying to pass information across to autistic children. As time goes on, if your kid is being taught sign language, you may have to learn sign language, too, to foster communication and help strengthen the bond between you. While studying your child, it is also important to figure out what evokes violent or destructive behavior in him. Try to understand why he throws tantrums and figure out a way to help him control those outbursts. Gently, but firmly, teach him ways to politely communicate his displeasure and let him understand that you will always be there to help him out any time he needs your assistance.

Finally, with the help of your child's pediatrician and his therapists, you should be able to figure out a special treatment plan that works for your child. You must keep in mind that you will be the one spending time with your child, and you are the one who is in the best position to choose from an available range of options based upon your personal assessments of your child's behavior. This is why it is important to make some tough choices and sacrifices to enable you to be around your child as much as possible. While discussing options with the healthcare experts, you must try to determine a treatment plan that will build on your child's specific interests, teach him or her simple tasks, actively engage his/her attention, help him/her inculcate good behaviors, and help enhance his/her social skills. It is also very important that you be an integral part of the design of his specific treatment plan, because you will be the one carrying out the bulk of the plan. It is therefore important for you to come to critical conclusions with your child's healthcare experts based on the characteristics you have observed in your child and for you to offer your counsel where their generalizations are coming in conflict with your personal knowledge. In short, watch your child closely, and use your observations to work with qualified medical personnel to help choose an efficient treatment plan for your boy or girl.

Finally, it is important for you, as the parent of an autistic child, to look for useful help and support for your child's growth. Information about financial, legal, and medical aid may be available online on official websites, but it is quite important for you to double-check information found from doubtful sources to prevent fraud or misinformation. A Federal Law in the United States, the Individuals with Disabilities Education Act, has been designed to help children with special needs attain their needed education from the right institutions. A special type of curriculum may need to be designed for your child to help hone his innate skills based on your observations; hence, you need to be an active part of the design process. The Individualized Education Plan helps you figure out the right path to be taken so that you may educate a particular autistic child and enhance his own growth and development.

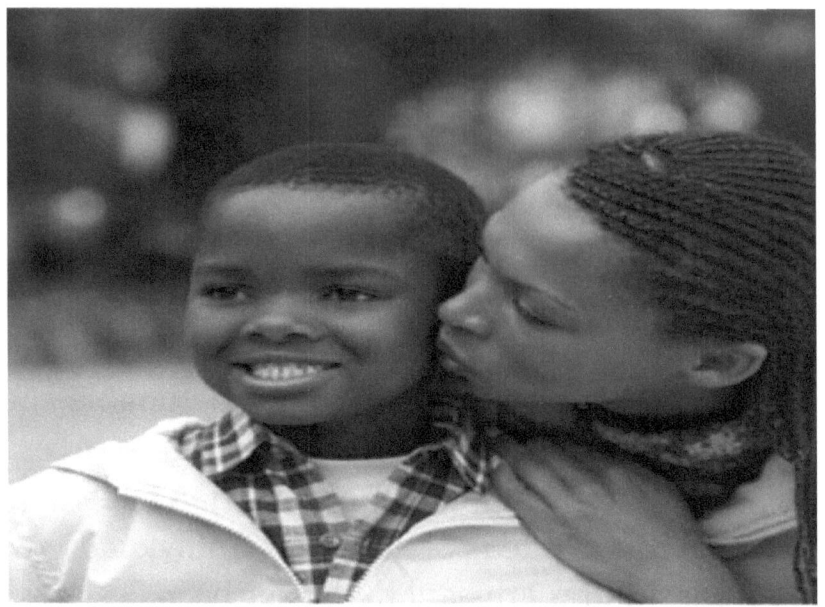

All in all, try your best to be your child's best friend. More than anyone else, he or she needs you.

CHAPTER 8: DEALING WITH DISABILITIES IN AFRICAN COUNTRIES AND COMMUNITIES IN THE DIASPORA

Being a person with special needs or taking care of a disabled person in a developing country can be very challenging. Factors such as local traditions and beliefs and intense alienation and stigmatization are some of the factors mitigating the well-being of autistic people in Africa and other communities in the diaspora.

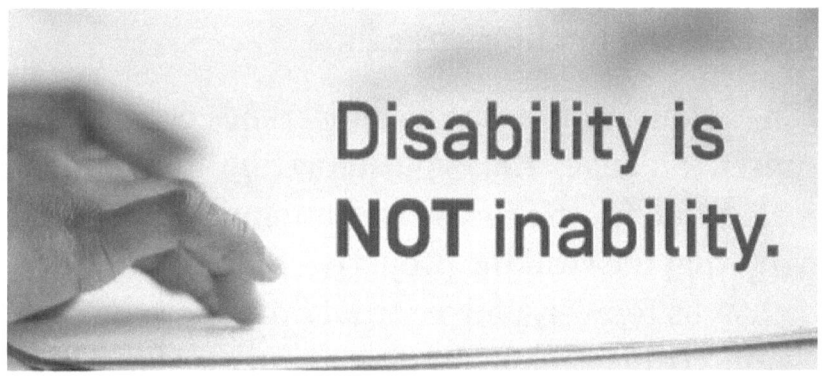

Karunga was a five-year-old born with autistic spectrum disorder. He was non-verbal, and he always had a sort of lost look in his eyes anytime he stared into space. He was born into a small fishing village in Rwanda, East Africa, where beliefs in ancient traditional practices only waxed stronger with time. He now sat in the middle of the village square, looking on with a keen interest that was masked by the lack of focus in his eyes as a huge flame burnt before him. Traditional dancers clad in traditional attires of raffia and banana leaves danced before him with all their strength to the feverish tune emanating from the huge village drum, which sounded any time there was need for a meeting or when there was an announcement to be made. As Karunga watched on, his mother sobbed at home whilst being comforted by the boy's father.

"We could pack our things and disappear with him, nobody would know!" Solange, Karunga's mother, wept, feeling totally distraught.

"They would notice our disappearance even before sunset, Solange. And you know the punishment meted out to offenders who attempt to abscond with what they call the property of the gods. They'd banish us forever, and we would never see our son again! Think about it deeply, my wife. Think deeply." Indogo, Karunga's father, said, at his wit's end.

Sibling Caregiver

"But I don't want him to grow up serving that useless old man…"

"Hush… be quiet, Solange! You don't want to be heard saying that. Walls have ears, you know. Now, put yourself together and let's get out there for the traditional rites. It's our duty, after all, even if it kills us to do it."

A teary, broken, and distraught Solange stood up and rested her frail form against her husband's muscular one. When Solange had first married Indogo, a brave hunter and farmer, about six years ago, she had been one of the most sought-after maidens in the village. All the eligible bachelors had jostled for her heart, bringing gifts ranging from antelopes, palm wine, and even expensive clothes for her all the time just to win her heart. Only one man had made her feel complete, however. Indogo wasn't rich, but he was very hard-working and sincere. He was very strong, too, and she had lost her heart to him when he saved her from a gang of village miscreants who rounded her up around dusk on the outskirts of the village. They wanted to have her for themselves, since they thought she was too proud to marry any man from the village. Indogo had arrived just as they had intended to begin their sacrilegious act. Strong as a horse and swift as a falcon, Indogo had beaten the daylights out of almost all of them before the last two ran back into the village, petrified, with their tails between their legs. Six months later, Solange had married her knight in shining armor.

Trouble, however, began in Paradise after Karunga's birth. The village had a long-standing rule: all 'abnormal' children, from children with physical disabilities to kids with cognitive disorders, were regarded as the property of the deities, and were not to be touched. On their fifth birthdays, a ceremony was to be held to induct them into the service of the deities. They would live in the chief priest's huge compound and be clad in red, with chalk used to mark their faces and cam wood smeared all over their bodies. They were naturally 'destined' to serve the gods all their lives, although their parents and family could come to visit them on specific occasions.

As Solange and Indogo arrived at the village square, the drums and dancing had reached a feverish pitch and the whole square seemed to be shaking from the earth's core. Karunga sat alone in front of the huge fire, scared and helpless. As Solange saw him, her precious child, she burst into tears again. Why did life have to be so unfair to her? What had she ever done to deserve this? A chicken was beheaded right above the fire by the chief priest, its blood dripping into the flames, while the rest of the blood was rubbed all over Karunga's body as the Priest ranted his incantations. Finally, he stopped and turned to face the crowd. The initiation was finished, and little Karunga was the property of the gods now. Solange screamed as they took him away, and she slowly slipped into unconsciousness.

In many African societies, a sort of spiritual meaning is attached to autism and various other cognitive and even physical disorders, like polio. Due to people's lack of exposure and understanding of these disabilities, people with autism are treated as outcasts and sometimes are even actually cast out of their communities to ward off what is seen as evil. In the urban cities however, a different sort of problem is usually faced by autistic children and their parents.

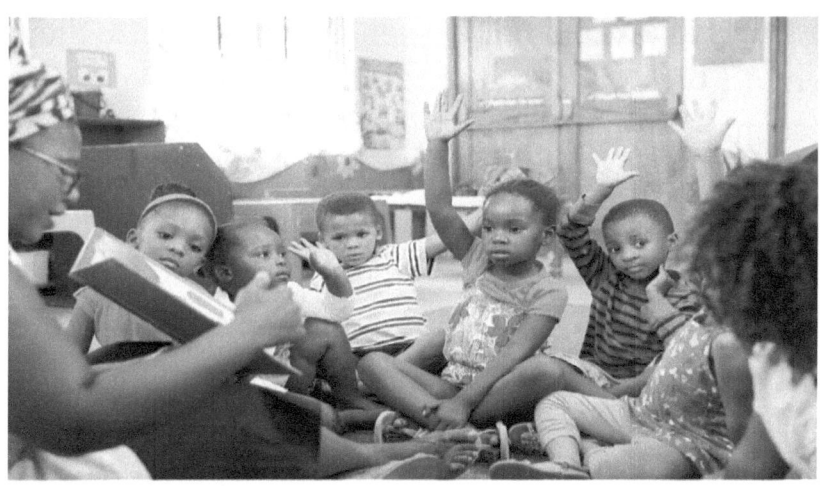

The first major challenge faced by autistic children and their parents in urban African society is quite similar to what is experienced in America and Europe: alienation. However, the alienation of these autistic children is stronger in Africa, because the stigmatization is reinforced by superstitious beliefs still held by many Africans. Some people have been known to take to their heels upon the sight of an autistic child. People need to understand that being autistic has no spiritual meaning whatsoever; it's just a medical condition, a cognitive disorder that can be contained and treated over time. What's even more appalling is that Africans who have migrated to the United States, or other western countries, bring with them the same misconceptions about people with disabilities. Within the African community in the US, there are many families with a child who has a disability that would rather be swallowed up in an earthquake than to be seen in public with their child. To help curb the menace of this stigmatization, campaigns and sensitization programs can and should be launched by the government and by not-for-profit organizations to help educate the public about the facts and truths surrounding autism and how autistic people actually need their help and support, not their discrimination.

Sibling Caregiver

Another major problem faced by most African societies in the fight against autism is the marked absence or intense shortage of appropriate medical facilities dedicated to the diagnosis and treatment of autistic patients. Research has also shown that the number of medical experts available who are actually well-grounded in the field of autism treatment and diagnostics are in fact very few. Therapists and psychological experts who can help set an autistic child on the road to recovery are also usually very difficult to find or afford for the average African. Due to this lack or shortage of appropriate medical facilities and personnel, most cases of autism in African societies are not given proper medical attention, and the kids are just watched as they struggle to cope with their lives. Parents usually play an active role in the gradual progress of their autistic children, but without appropriate medical attention, most of these kids barely get better over time. Some privileged children may be lucky enough to get access to quality medical care, but these facilities are usually expensive, and the percentage of children who actually gain access to these facilities is usually only a tiny fraction of the autistic population. The government and NGOs can work together, and grants and loans may be sought from international organizations like the Paris Club, the World Bank, or the International Monetary Fund to build well-equipped healthcare centers to cater to the needs of the African autistic population. Loans and grants may also be sought from foreign governments to aid in this cause. If an African country can afford it, however, the government should try to apportion a significant percentage of its budget to healthcare, and a large percentage of this figure should be dedicated to research on autism and construction of healthcare facilities to promote the welfare and well-being of autistic children.

Closely related to the inadequacy of appropriate medical facilities for autism treatment is the almost complete absence of social service centers to help cater to the needs of autistic persons and other people with chronic cognitive deficiencies in their local communities. Most African communities, even in urban cities, lack local social service centers, and most caregivers usually find themselves stuck in a rut when it comes to finding help and information related to autism in their local communities. African countries need to establish a solid, efficient social service and welfare network to help cater to the needs of autistic people and other people in their society generally. Funding should be directed towards the establishment of social services centers in major regions, and with time, more social services centers can be established to address the needs of people at the grassroots level.

Closely related to the absence of quality public social services is the unavailability of resources, such as financial aid and respite care, for caregivers of autistic people. In the United States and other first-world countries, facilities have been put in place to help ease the financial strain on sibling and informal caregivers and to ensure access by autistic people to the best medical care. In African countries, however, health insurance is not a capacity possessed by the majority of the population, and most people actually opt for self-medication when it comes to common diseases like malaria, cough, and even typhoid fever. Facilities offering quality treatment to autistic children are few, and these facilities usually charge a lot for their services. A huge percentage of the autistic population cannot afford these expensive medical fees, and due to the absence of financial aid or support from the government, these autistic kids fail to get the treatment they need to develop mentally. Respite care is another social service that is almost non-existent in most African countries. Respite care is when a caregiver invites a volunteer or a dedicated public service worker over to help care for his or her loved one while he/she takes time off to avoid intense stress and burnout.

Due to the absence of respite care and other social service facilities, most caregivers face intense stress and burnout in the discharge of their duties as caregivers. This leads to rampant cases of caregiver abuse, in which the care recipients get severely brutalized in some cases. Intense stress can also lead to severe health conditions such as depression and high blood pressure in most caregivers. The fact that quality medical care is not readily available to treat even the depressed and hypertensive caregivers makes matters terribly worse. Stress among African caregivers is usually sky high, because they rarely get the help they need due to the superstitious beliefs attached to autism by most members of the society. This intense stigmatization of autistic people by even friends and family members makes getting the much-needed help of caring for caregivers' care recipients very difficult, and it makes the quality of care received by the autistic child completely inadequate. The lack of other stress-relieving facilities, such as adult day care centers and residential homes for people with special needs, also makes the stress faced by African caregivers even more intense.

The future of many autistic African children is in jeopardy. This is because the educational sectors of most African societies have not even been able to effectively finance basic education for regular average kids to a satisfactory extent, let alone talk of building and maintaining enough special educational facilities for the children with learning disabilities. The scarcity of special education centers and the absence of programs like the Individualized Educational Plan make the quality of education received by autistic children appalling. Most autistic children must cope with going to the same government-funded schools as their non-autistic counterparts, where the quality of education is usually nothing to write home about even for them. Under these conditions, autistic children who have challenges retaining information in the first place learn virtually nothing and may find it difficult to proceed to junior high at the end of their primary education, since they have barely learnt anything at all through their years in grade school. The education and health sectors need to work together to put special educational facilities in place specifically designed to cater to the needs of autistic children to ensure their mental development, and to enable them to grow up to become assets, and not liabilities, to African society at large.

Finally, the federal governments in African countries need to work together with not-for-profit organizations and other developed countries to enact laws to help foster the well-being of the African autistic population. These laws should include provisions to help ensure the availability of quality healthcare and financial assistance to autistic children and to help provide quality educational services to autistic children, even if it has to be at a cost. Educating the autistic population is very important, and even if the government can't provide structures to house special educational centers for autistic children yet, sections of existing schools can be dedicated to the education of children with special needs. This, however, needs to be done carefully to avoid segregation, and as soon as experts deem it fit to do so, these autistic children may be gradually integrated into the traditional educational system. To solve the problem of shortage of medical experts, attractive remuneration should be attached to the roles of medical experts treating autism in public hospitals, and investors, both local and foreign, should be encouraged to establish healthcare facilities to help foster the well-being of the autistic population through the creation of favorable policies and attractions, such as lower taxes. To help ease the stress of caregivers, a sort of government agency may be established to help cater to the needs of caregivers and care recipients. The journey to quality care for the African autistic population is a long one, but if all the stakeholders come together to work with the government, superior quality care can be achieved in the long run.

CHAPTER 9: WHERE DO WE GO FROM HERE?

When we examine the structure of society today, it is easy to discover that there is actually no solid lifetime plan available for autistic people. Except for those autistic people who have superior mental abilities, like some people with Asperger's syndrome, who can focus intensely on one line of thought to execute difficult tasks at mind-blowing speeds, and those with other disorders on the autistic spectrum which make patients in one way or another exceptional (art, music, or dance), who can confidently go into the world to perform even better than their counterparts, most autistic patients face the danger of a future full of uncertainties. Even though many first-world countries have worked hard to put in place facilities to help autistic people develop their innate skills and to help caregivers relieve stress, the same cannot be said for third-world countries. The final, most scathing truth is that after autistic people all over the world finish their education, they are all faced with the challenge of how to gain suitable employment to help them earn a decent income for themselves. The truth is that most highly demanding business environments find it difficult to employ autistic people, due to the complex nature of the jobs there. How, then, can we advance the cause of autistic people in today's society, and how can autistic people be effectively integrated into society? How can the quality of care available to autistic patients in third-world countries be improved upon? What are the roles that governments, corporate bodies, and individuals have to play in helping autistic people all over the world? Where do we go from here?

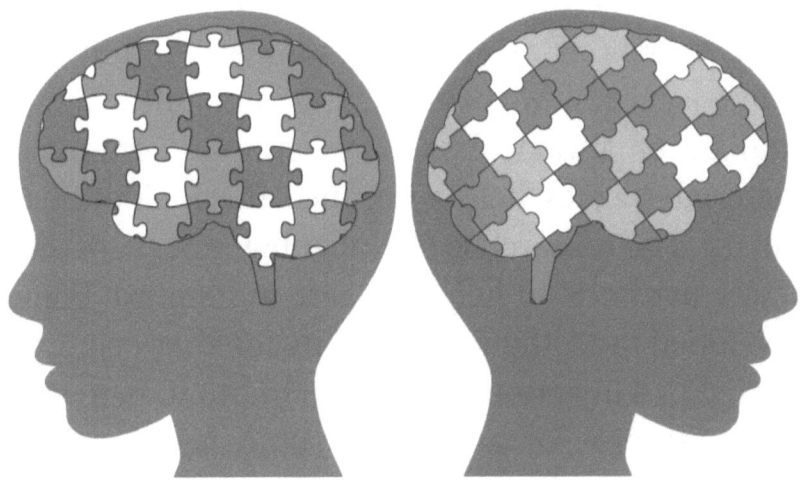

First of all, the government has a huge role to play in working towards the better treatment of autistic people and in funding research that aims at helping autistic people live better, more normal lives. The government needs to invest more in research to mitigate the effects of autism, or maybe even to cure the disorder. According to research today, gut bacteria and mice who exhibit autism-like behavior have been very helpful in studying the genetic transfer of autistic traits. Researchers at the Baylor College of Medicine in Texas have been studying the effects that gut bacteria in expectant mothers have on neurologically active compounds that have been found to alter cognitive functioning and behavioral patterns. The doctors have since managed to add a specific species of bacteria to the guts of the mice. The new species have been found to help lower the number of autistic mice given birth to among a selected population that has otherwise been witnessing a significantly higher number of autistic births. In simple terms, the bacterial species help to reduce the incidence of autism. The research is still ongoing, but every day, newer methods to help mitigate autism are being developed, and the future keeps looking brighter. Methyl B12 injections have been found to help ease the symptoms of autism in some people. Gene mutations in only peripheral sensory neurons have also been found to be influence the symptoms that comprise autism. All in all, the government needs to channel more energy towards research to help find a cure for autism spectrum disorder, or at least to find better scientific methods to treat autism and give autistic patients a better life.

Available social service facilities could also be improved upon to help bring respite care and surgical procedures within the reach of the average autistic patient anywhere in the world. More financial aid can be put in place to help ease the financial strain on informal caregivers, and caregivers need to be more sensitized about how to properly care for their patients. With the aid of research, easier and more effective methods of caring for care recipients while caregivers attend to other tasks can also be developed. Available medical facilities also need to be improved upon, new specialists need to be trained, and those currently available should undergo further education to keep them abreast of new discoveries in the study of autism.

Individuals, corporate organizations, and not-for-profit organizations can also do a lot to help autistic people. Corporate organizations can work with the government to help make social services available in regions where they aren't yet. Not-for-profit organizations can stage more campaigns to educate people about autism while also organizing charity dinners to help build adult day care centers and residential care homes, and, finally, special educational institutions. There is a lot to do for everybody, but together, we can all help make the world a better and warmer place for every autistic child out there. What's important is that we all play our part.

ABOUT THE AUTHOR

OB Nwaogbe is a political commentator, producer, the voice for social injustice, equal rights for women, immigration, and an advocate for people who can't speak for themselves.

As a television producer and news reporter for the past 10yrs, OB has had the priviedge of covering stories that appeal to an international audience. Her empolyment in the field of broadcast journalism spans various media entities, including NBC 4 Washington DC, PBS, Fema Recovery Channel, DCTV, Montgomery Community Media, and the United Negro Colleg Fund Special Programs TV. She is the founder of The News with OB, an online news magazine show that covers current affairs, politics, and news happening in the local community and around the world.

REFRENCES

Informal Caregiver Law and Legal Definition: https://definitions.uslegal.com/i/informal-caregiver/

Caregiver Abuse Law and Legal Definition: https://definitions.uslegal.com/c/caregiver-abuse/

Social services: https://en.wikipedia.org/wiki/Social_services

Adult daycare center: https://en.wikipedia.org/wiki/Adult_daycare_center

Care Act 2014: http://www.legislation.gov.uk/ukpga/2014/23/enacted

30 Resources to Help Caregivers: https://www.senioradvisor.com/blog/2017/04/30-resources-to-help-caregivers/

UNSPOKEN WORDS: WORKS BY AUTISTIC ARTISTS: http://42maple.org/project/unspoken-words-works-by-autistic-artists/

INDEX

acceptance, 31, 33, 39, 41, 94
autism, 13, 23, 89, 91, 94, 96, 98, 100, 101, 103, 119, 120, 121, 122, 124, 126, 129, 131
Autism, 1, 94, 103
Book a ride, 67
CARE Act, 76, 77
caregiver, iii, 1, 5, 6, 7, 8, 9, 10, 14, 15, 16, 17, 18, 19, 21, 23, 25, 26, 27, 28, 29, 30, 31, 32, 33, 34, 36, 38, 39, 40, 43, 44, 45, 47, 48, 50, 52, 53, 54, 55, 56, 57, 59, 60, 61, 62, 63, 64, 66, 68, 70, 74, 76, 77, 78, 80, 81, 83, 86, 94, 98, 101, 123, 124, 134
caregiver abuse, 18, 36, 44, 45, 52, 54, 55, 56, 81, 124
community living, 17, 21, 28, 32, 51
Companionship services, 63
day care centers, 21, 69, 70, 71, 72, 73, 74, 124, 131
emotional stress, 19, 33, 35, 45, 55, 67
Ethnicity, 82
financial assistance, 25, 26, 28, 74, 85, 126
healthcare, 28
Housekeeping services, 63
LGBT, 84, 85
Meal prep services, 64
Medicaid, 25, 67
non-profit organizations, 22, 24, 51, 58, 61
parents, iii, 1, 12, 13, 87, 89, 94, 100, 101, 118, 119, 120
physical stress, 18, 49, 67
religions, 82

resources, 5, 41, 46, 48, 51, 56, 58, 60, 61, 80, 81, 86, 123, 134
respite services, 28, 46
sexual orientation, 84, 85
sibling caregiver, 6, 14, 15, 16, 25, 48, 55
stress, 7, 18, 19, 24, 25, 27, 44, 45, 49, 54, 55, 56, 60, 62, 63, 68, 74, 80, 81, 82, 93, 94, 97, 123, 124, 126, 128

www.ingramcontent.com/pod-product-compliance
Lightning Source LLC
Chambersburg PA
CBHW030007190526
45157CB00014B/1014